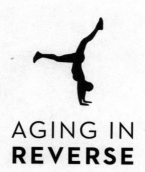

AGING IN
REVERSE

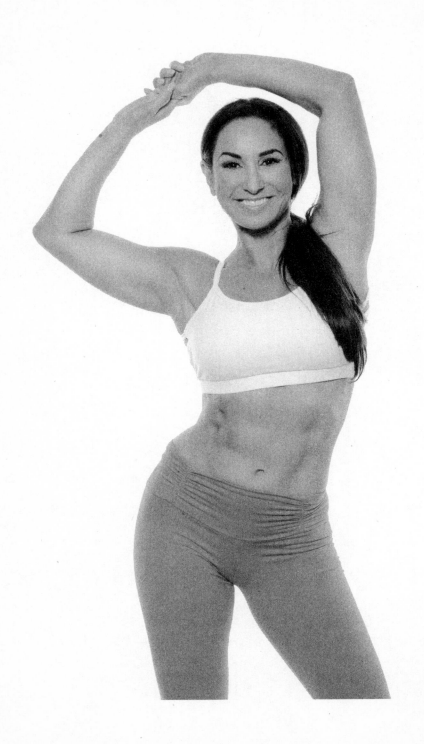

AGING IN
REVERSE

The Easy **10-DAY PLAN** *to*
Change Your State, Plan Your Plate,
Love Your Weight

Natalie Jill

Da Capo
LIFE
LONG

Copyright © 2019 by Natalie Jill
Cover design by Alex Camlin
Cover image by Noel Daganta
Cover copyright © 2019 Hachette Book Group, Inc.

Hachette Book Group supports the right to free expression and the value of copyright. The purpose of copyright is to encourage writers and artists to produce the creative works that enrich our culture.

The scanning, uploading, and distribution of this book without permission is a theft of the author's intellectual property. If you would like permission to use material from the book (other than for review purposes), please contact permissions@hbgusa.com. Thank you for your support of the author's rights.

Da Capo Press
Hachette Book Group
1290 Avenue of the Americas, New York, NY 10104
www.dacapopress.com
@DaCapoPress

Printed in the United States of America

First Edition: May 2019

Published by Da Capo Press, an imprint of Perseus Books, LLC, a subsidiary of Hachette Book Group, Inc. The Da Capo Press name and logo is a trademark of the Hachette Book Group.

The Hachette Speakers Bureau provides a wide range of authors for speaking events. To find out more, go to www.hachettespeakersbureau.com or call (866) 376-6591.

The publisher is not responsible for websites (or their content) that are not owned by the publisher.

Exercise photographs by Lauren Reid; all other photographs by Natalie Minn.
Print book interior design by Cynthia Young at Sagecraft.

Library of Congress Cataloging-in-Publication Data has been applied for.

ISBNs: 978-0-7382-3532-5 (hardcover), 978-0-7382-3533-2 (ebook)

LSC-C

10 9 8 7 6 5 4 3 2 1

To my husband, Brooks, and my daughter, Penelope.
Thanks for your push to always better myself and for helping
me to know that thoughts always become our reality.

Contents

PART 3
Love Your Weight   249

· ·

Taking Unprocessed up a Notch

It doesn't matter where you're at—
it's where you want to go.

I thought I was doing everything right. I was running a successful fitness and nutrition business, and in my midforties, I was in the most amazing shape of my life.

And then I tanked.

It became really noticeable en route to an all-day workout shoot in Miami, but it actually had been building up for some time before that. I already had some mild disc bulge in my lower back, as many people my age do, but I thought I could ignore it and keep on going as if nothing had changed. My ego got in the way of getting real with my body's needs to prevent the disaster that happened.

At the workout shoot, my brain was telling me to slow down, but I wouldn't listen. I was doing some high-impact moves that I normally don't do, which was not helping. I *knew* not to do those moves in my situation. My "normal" mild back pain started escalating to horrible back pain, worse than I even experienced during labor. It was by far the most pain I had ever been in, a dull pain that kept getting worse. But I didn't complain about it and kept pushing through.

To this day I don't know how I did it, but I got through the day, went to sleep, and when I woke up the next morning, the pain in my back was gone. However, when I got out of bed, something was wrong with my right leg through to my piriformis (one of the glute muscles). It was sort of heavy, like it was asleep and lagging behind me. It was still working, but it felt as if it wasn't listening to my brain. There was a total delay in movement. I thought I must have just strained something and it would heal on its own.

As I walked sluggishly through the airport to fly back to California, my leg continued to feel heavy and delayed. Through the flight, it kept getting worse, to the point that it almost felt like I was getting paralyzed. This continued for three days. Still, I thought that I'd just pulled something and that it would get better.

But it didn't get better. The pain in my piriformis went into my hip and lower back. Going from sitting to standing became almost impossible. In tears I called an orthopedic surgeon friend, and he told me to get an MRI right away. I did what he said, and the doctor showed me that the disc bulge had completely ruptured and was wrapped around my spinal cord, which was impinging on my sciatic nerve. That's why I was losing feeling in my right leg. He warned me it was going to keep getting worse unless I removed the ruptured mass.

The doctor immediately got me in with a specialty surgeon. The surgeon looked at my MRI, and I was in surgery two days later. He explained to me that if I were to let it go any longer, I would have permanent damage to my right leg. He told me that the foot drop I was experiencing—meaning my foot would literally drag while I walked—could become permanent. The surgery was successful, though my surgeon told me that it was one of the largest ruptures he had ever seen. I haven't regained my full balance yet, but I'm 90 percent back, still moving forward, and grateful that no lasting damage was done.

Could I have prevented the ruptured disc? I don't know. But I do know that I had been in denial. I thought maybe my symptoms and the 10 pounds that came with them were simply aging or my hormones. Yes, it's true that our body doesn't quite bounce back the way it does when we're younger. But

I know from myself and the many clients I've worked with that we can be at the top of our game at any point in our lives. Those of us who don't experience pain as we age are typically using our body in a functional way. This means our body works as a unit, without imbalances or weak links. Our core (that whole middle section) and our body move how they are supposed to. With my abs and strong-looking core appearing on multiple magazine covers, I always considered myself one of those people!

But somewhere along the way, I started to ignore pain's warning signs. I was pushing myself in ways that weren't serving me anymore. I knew that I needed to spend more time on my warm-ups and doing the right moves to keep my body in balance—stretching out my hip flexors, firing my glutes, and keeping the muscles I couldn't see (the stabilizer muscles) strong so they could continue to do their job of supporting the muscles I *could* see. Looking back, I believe that my six-pack abs were a false sense of security for some of the deeper issues I had going on with my body. I knew that I needed more rest and time between travel and working out, and I needed to put more effort into staying hydrated and properly nourished. If I were consulting with a client, I would have told her not to wear heels all the time—that being fashionable was outweighing functional and smart for her! After the surgery, I did some soul searching. But not before wondering whether my career was over. The workout wasn't the cause of the ruptured disc. Not taking care of my body and not doing what I knew to do was the cause. I had so many limiting beliefs—what I call self-imposed stops—that I believed I was doomed, my business went downhill, and my relationships started to crumble. My stress level was getting out of control and it seemed as if everything was going horribly wrong. *How could this have happened to me? Should I even be teaching fitness anymore?* I wondered. *How could I call myself a fitness expert and do something so stupid! Maybe age really is an issue. Maybe I'm not good enough to be doing what I do.*

But soon enough, I caught myself, and instead of turning to excuses, instead of hitting rock bottom again, I delved deeper. I learned that if I had honed in on an anti-inflammatory diet and focused on corrective circuits and workouts, I could have taken the disc out of the equation and all that came after might not have happened. And most important, I learned that changing my state of mind could serve me powerfully and help me avoid this happening again. This newfound knowledge became a new reset for my life and my career and the inspiration for this book. I became committed to helping others avoid the mistakes I made.

Looking Back

About two decades ago, I had been diagnosed with celiac disease, a condition in which a person is unable to digest gluten. This was before everyone started talking about gluten intolerance and it became popular to be on a gluten-free diet. So, I had to do a lot of research and figure out what to do for myself. To cut out the gluten, I had to eliminate most processed foods. But as awareness and technology advanced, more and more gluten-free replacement foods, such as pizza, bread, and cookies, were becoming available, and convenience won out. Why? Because, at the time, my life was spiraling out of control. I was a new mom, recently divorced, working too much, and suffering the effects of an economic downturn. I became depressed and gained 60 pounds. My diet was built around gluten-free processed carbs and grains. Corn, oatmeal, cheese, mashed potatoes, and ice cream were staples in my diet.

Something had to change so I could get my life back, and I knew what I had to do. I remembered what I talked about with my Fortune 500 clients: creating a vision, declaring an intention, setting goals, and eliminating self-imposed stops. I had to go back to the vision board and set new goals. I had to decide that I was ready to shift again and that failure would not be an option. And, most of all, I had to unprocess my diet again.

Long story short, it worked! I turned my problems into opportunities. I lost all the extra weight, and not only that, I became a fitness model at age thirty-nine and was featured on the cover of several magazines, including *Woman's World*! I found my true calling: helping others to become the best version of themselves. I became a Licensed Master Sports Nutritionist, and millions of people have been enjoying my fitness videos and lifestyle nutrition plans. Even more people have lost weight and gotten into shape with the program and recipes I shared in my best-selling first book, *Natalie Jill's 7-Day Jump Start*. I was recognized as one of the top fitness influencers in the world by *Forbes* and *Greatist*. I was changing lives and having fun doing it!

Looking Forward

Nearly a decade later, with pain as a wake-up call, I remembered what I did to get where I am today, and I took stock. I realized that every time I hit a setback, the first thing that had to shift was not a new technology, gimmick, or diet plan, but *me*. I had to change my state. What got me through every hurdle I'd encountered was deciding that there was a possibility of getting out of it. What could I do to shift my mind-set? What did I need to start doing differently? What did I need to do daily to step into a powerful, confident me? So many of us stay comfortable with what we know, but in reality we need to constantly check in with ourselves and make adjustments if we want to stay true to our vision.

To change my state, I had to meet my body where it was. I owed it to my audience to be authentic with them. I told them what I was going through so they could learn from my experience. I admitted that I didn't know everything and that I was getting help to figure it all out. And this resonated and landed with so many! I couldn't believe it. What was embarrassing for me to share became the connection between my audience and me. They wanted more. *Muscle & Fitness Hers* magazine even put me on their cover and did a feature article on me after my comeback.

As I recovered from the surgery, I put my ego aside and sought the help of experts, including a couple of physical therapists, a few trainers specializing in corrective exercises, and coaches to help me with emotional intelligence and more. I became an education magnet. I wanted to learn how to prevent this from happening to me again, and I wanted to teach other people how to avoid getting into a similar situation. I shifted my workouts to include a huge restorative focus with a goal of healing and preventing future pain. I'll share these moves with you later in the book.

Understanding what exactly inflammation is and the link between inflammation and pain became my mission. Inflammation is the body's reaction to stress—stress from the environment, diet, or invaders and infections. Think about when you cut your skin: the area gets hot and red for a while, but eventually the cut is healed. This is short-term inflammation, and it's a good thing. But when inflammation goes on too long, it's no longer helpful. Your body is constantly trying to heal itself from the damage you've done, but it's just not working, so the inflammation never goes away. Prolonged inflammation is tied to nearly every chronic disease, including heart disease, cancer, Alzheimer's disease, and diabetes.

I came to the conclusion that to get the inflammation down, I had to not only keep eating unprocessed foods, but to take unprocessed up a notch. I had to plan my plate differently by removing inflammation-triggering foods and adding even more veggies, probiotic-rich fermented foods, and anti-inflammatory superfoods. But targeting the immediate pain was only a part of the healing. Quelling the flames of inflammation is our ticket to aging in reverse. (This can be especially important when we are going through peri-menopause and menopause; I'll talk about this more on pages 126 to 134.)

Introducing the Transformation Triangle

From my newfound realization, the Transformation Triangle was born. The Triangle's three-point plan—Change Your State, Plan Your Plate, and Love Your Weight—pulls together my proven tools for an unprocessed lifestyle that will serve you at every point of your life. It's not just about weight loss. Weight loss can be short lived, and it can fool us because it's only part of the picture. You may think you are headed in the right direction, only to realize your clothes aren't fitting you better and you aren't feeling better. You are still in pain, less than confident, and your moods and energy aren't at 100 percent. But when you engage all three points of the Transformation Triangle, everything shifts. You feel better in your skin and you get stronger. Your skin starts glowing, your focus improves, and your driving core motivator kicks in so you keep improving every day. You'll understand what you need to do to lose or maintain your weight, clear your brain, keep hot flashes in check, recharge, and get your mojo back. That's what I mean by aging in reverse! And you won't just lose the weight but you'll come to a place of loving your weight.

But first things first. The entire first part of the book, Change Your State, is dedicated to mind-set. Don't skip over it. Why? *Because every single one of my clients has told me that they couldn't have done the work without changing their state.* When you read through the transformation stories that Mira (page 47), Nicole (page 54), Susana (page 91), Yulanda (page 139),

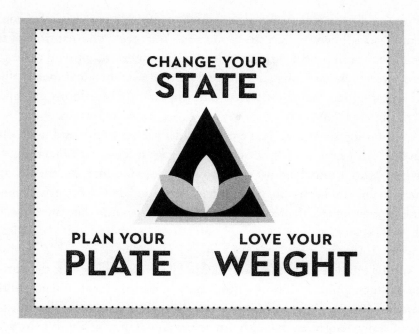

CHANGE YOUR
STATE

PLAN YOUR
PLATE

LOVE YOUR
WEIGHT

Amanda (page 246), and Terri (page 276) have shared, you'll understand just what I mean!

As we get older, we definitely need to get more serious about how we are eating. What we could have gotten away with years ago may not work for us now. But what keeps us stuck is not our body but our mind. My 10 Tools to Change Your State has helped women of all ages, shapes, and sizes get on track and meet their health and fitness goals. It starts with creating a vision. Then, you make a firm decision to follow through, breaking through self-imposed stops with the force of a superhero. You might be going through menopause and believe that those extra 10 pounds, forgetfulness, and memory loss are inevitable because that's what everyone tells you. Turn that self-imposed stop around by finding others who have learned to stay fit and clear-headed as they age. Changing your state includes finding your driving core motivator—what truly motivates you to make changes that last—creating new habits and routines, adding as much good as you can, and connecting with people who are on the same path. Only then does your transformation truly begin!

After you've changed your state, you're ready to plan your plate. You're open to eating in a way that serves you *now*. You may be in that time of life when your hormones are shifting, a time that is not exactly a friend to weight loss or even to maintaining your shape. With a slower metabolism and affinity for storing fat, there's simply no room in your diet for foods that aren't nourishing. It's time to make unprocessed even more important.

It's common sense for anyone concerned with her health and well-being to avoid highly processed options, such as sugary snacks, crackers, chips, and anything with a mile-long list of impossible-to-pronounce ingredients, but it's especially crucial at this time. When you're in the throes of perimenopause or menopause, they can be especially toxic—not just because of calories, but because of how your body breaks down these foods. We'll learn more about that later.

And by eliminating some foods that may have served you in the past—such as dairy, grains, and beans—but are now causing bloat, inflammation, and mind fog, omitting sugar from your diet completely, and following ten days of supercharged eating with my new menu plan, you'll find your body can't help but get back on track. Bolstered with a new way of looking at your body and exercising in the final section, Love Your Weight, you will learn to progress and challenge yourself in ways that work for you at any time of life. You might be experiencing aches and pains you think are a natural part of aging. You might think your days of working out are over. This is just a self-imposed stop! You can learn how to do corrective exercises, just as I did, to get out of the pain. As you work the Transformation Triangle, pain and inflammation will decrease, mood swings will stabilize, and you'll win your confidence back. You just have to believe that you can do it.

Some of my clients have sustained injuries that put limits on their workouts. But when they set their mind to it and planned their plate differently, they started losing weight and were able to build up their energy. The pain that was stopping them from working out lessened or went away. They were able to become more active and have even more powerful transformations. In short, what you think and what you eat has the power to change your whole body and your whole life!

As you get older, you may feel like everything is a challenge. I get it. But I'm not here to validate excuses. I'm here to help you find solutions! There's no good reason to let age or changing hormones become a self-imposed stop. Age forty-five, fifty-five, or sixty-five, and older can look completely different from what you expect. Educating yourself through hormonal changes is one of the key tools to staying healthy, sexy, and fit through what otherwise could be a roller-coaster ride.

People are always shocked when I tell them my age (forty-seven as I write this book), but a numerical age can mean many different things. Because they see me on the cover of magazines, they want to know what my secret is. It's an inside job. Age, health, and happiness start with mind-set, and from there, planning your plate and loving your weight will flow naturally. The Transformation Triangle got me through a major hurdle in my life, and it will give you the tools for aging in reverse so you can be your best, youngest-looking, and youngest-feeling self at every point in yours.

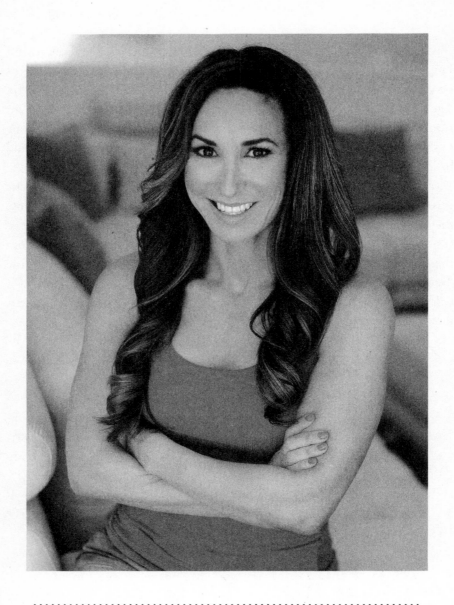

If you follow a diet or workout plan without changing your state, you will not get lasting results and it will become easy to give up. If you don't believe it's going to work, it won't.

PART 1

Change Your State:
10 Steps to Shift Your Mind-set

The most important thing I've learned through both my personal coaching practice and my own transformation is that if you want your body to change, *you've got to start with your mind*. My work has never been just about diet and fitness. The first priority is to ditch the head games to create a body and life you love. Changing your state means uncovering the beliefs that got you where you are now and replacing them with new, positive thoughts with the power to propel you toward loving your body and your life.

If you follow a diet or workout plan without changing your state, you will not get lasting results and it will become easy to give up. If you don't believe it's going to work, it won't. That's why changing your state is at the top of the Transformation Triangle. Promise me that before you head to the meal plan or even start your shopping list, that you will make a commitment to do this for yourself. Changing your state is that missing link that makes transformation possible.

I can get you to results by doing a hard sell of the meal plan and hovering over you to do the workouts. However, once you are on your own, those results won't last unless you shift your state. When you shift your state to become a powerful, confident person on a mission to better yourself, results keep coming and fat loss lasts. So much will start to open up for you—not only your health and weight, but clarity and purpose to start living out your bigger vision and realize your goals.

You can't get results that last without changing your state. It's like a tripod. If you remove State from the Transformation Triangle, it will fall over, and Plate and Weight are doomed for failure. You need all three, and your state comes first. Once your mind is all in, everything starts to shift, and you'll be ready to scale down the sides of the Triangle and embrace my healthy eating plan and workout routines. And if you find yourself coming up with excuses, remember that *everyone* has excuses. It just comes down to whether you use them or not.

Many of us are familiar with the saying "Where the mind goes the body will always follow." I like to add "and with that your vision becomes your reality." When your mind is in the right place, it's a lot easier to get your body in good shape. And when your mind and body are in alignment, transformation is not only possible, but absolutely happens. You become unstoppable!

The following ten steps will help you establish and maintain a mind-set so you can get the results you want.

Step 1

Get Clear on Your Vision

If you don't know where you want to go, how can you get there? I want you to take some time to truly visualize how you want to feel, then imagine what your day and life would look like if you were living your goals. How would you be spending your time? Who would you be with? Where would you be living and what would your schedule look like? What would you be eating, and how would you be moving your body? Set clear intentions, make a declaration, and commit.

Putting it down on paper is the best way I know of getting clear on your vision. A picture is worth a thousand words—multiply that with intention and you create a mind map with happiness your destination. In my last book, *7-Day Jump Start: Unprocess Your Diet*, I talked a lot about creating a vision board as a way of getting real with how you want to feel and what you want to manifest in your life.

Are you thinking the vision board concept is too New Agey or hokey for you? And what does it have to do about eating well and getting in shape? Just commit to making one, and I promise you the results will speak for themselves! After I put together my first vision board, everything in my life changed for the better. I pasted photos of fit women, healthy food, and happy scenes—what I wanted my life to look like. And then, I started to work in that direction. The results? Now I have a career in fitness and in nutrition. I'm happy. I remarried. Even the smaller details manifested: my husband and

I bought the same model and make of car I randomly cut and pasted, and we moved to a home overlooking a beautiful golf course, just like the one on my vision board. *Eight years after making my first vision board, every single thing I put on it has come true.* And I've been making a new one every single year.

Having goals without vision always falls short. When you fine-tune your vision and take a good look at it—as you can do daily with your vision board—your goals go from possibility to reality. You grab the opportunity to be the best possible you.

If you've never made a vision board before, now's the time! If you made one in the past—after reading my first book or while you were working one of my other programs—it's time to start cutting and pasting again. I make a new vision board every year, and I recommend that you do this, too. You can use a vision board at any point in your life.

As you go through images and search for what you really want at this time in your life, your current goals will become clear. Healthy . . . youthful . . . energized . . . cut out words and images to match your vision and watch them manifest. Let yourself really get into it and allow your feelings and emotions to come to the surface. You are making your vision board for you, not anyone else. What drums up your emotions? Where do you feel sadness? Happiness? Hope? As you rummage through the magazines, note where you are inspired. What makes you deflated? Notice it all. It is amazing what you can uncover about yourself while creating a vision board. It is not uncommon to hear from clients that things they "weren't even aware of that they wanted" showed up. The possibilities really are endless.

Exercise:
Make a Vision Board

1. Grab a stack of magazines—whatever's visually appealing to you, such as magazines on vacation, fitness, or cooking. Use *real* magazines, not photos from Pinterest or other online sources. The very act of rummaging through the magazines will get your eyes to stop and gravitate toward things you might not have expected.

2. Grab a poster board, scissors, and glue or tape. Naturally, my boards are usually hot pink!

3. Cut out images, words, and headlines that you are drawn to.

4. Glue stick or tape what you've cut out to the board and add color—and even a little sparkle—if you like.

5. Hang your vision board in a place where you'll see it every day. You could even take a picture of it and make it the screensaver on your phone or computer! Take time to imagine you are *in* your vision board. What would you be doing as that person? How would that person be spending her days? What would she be eating? Who would be in her life? What would she *not* be doing? For example, my first vision board had views of the ocean. I would look at the images as if I were living with an ocean view. I knew that person would see the water every day, so I made it a point to drive by or walk near the ocean as often as possible. And the first place I moved to had a panoramic ocean view!

Now that you've made your vision board (wasn't that fun?) you can't just hang it up and sit around watching TV. You still have to take action! Think about what you can do to manifest your dreams. Read books, listen to talks, and meet with people who can facilitate your vision. Until you get where you want to be, keep looking at your vision board. (And once you're there, continue to look at it for reinforcement.) Remember where you want to go, and your vision board will be there to remind you to take action.

BONUS: Have a vision board party! Invite a few friends over and instruct everyone to grab her favorite color board and a stack of magazines. Try asking salons or doctors' offices for magazines from their waiting room that they are ready to get rid of.

LEARN TO POWERFULLY SAY NO

Are you someone who likes to say yes to everything? Are you always putting other people's priorities before yours? You might think you're doing the right thing, but in actuality you've got to get a little "self-ish" so you can best show up for both yourself and everyone else. When we constantly tend to other people's needs before our own, we are not being the best parent, the best spouse, the best friend, or the best employee. By saying yes to everyone else first, we put our vision last. Part of changing your mind-set is understanding that you are equally important. Learning to powerfully say no will serve you well. Before saying yes to anything, I ask myself, *Does this fit in with the vision for my life?* and *Would the person living in my vision board do this?* Learning this discernment is absolutely critical for achieving not just your diet and fitness goals but everything you want to accomplish in your life. Here are some tips for getting there:

Get grounded. Think about a day in which you did everything you wanted to do and felt powerful while doing it. A day in which you felt patient, present, calm, focused, and confident. A day in which everything just seemed to work in your favor. Maybe you were off from work, so you slept in, made yourself a leisurely breakfast, worked out, and had lunch with a friend. How did you feel? Did you have more energy? Were you happy? Maybe you had an epiphany about work or your fitness routine. How can you find this same type of inspiration in your everyday life?

How can you shift your space so you can be fully present for other people but still have time for you? How can you ground yourself daily in your vision and intentions so that you can be a better, more purposeful you?

Get laser focused. We all have the same amount of time in a day. You can't just magically find more time, but what you can do is restructure your day to shift out things that aren't serving you. Make a list of what you do on your average day. If you find this difficult, note down everything you do today. When I did this exercise, I made some surprising discoveries: I was spending a lot more time on social media and checking e-mail than I had thought. So, I made a decision to take e-mail off my phone and schedule an hour in my day for checking e-mail undistracted, which ended up saving me a lot of time. Check your list for sneaky gaps where you're wasting time or doing things that aren't helping with your goals. Could that extra hour on Facebook be better spent making healthy snacks for the week? Make decisions to free up time for the things you really need to get accomplished so that you can get laser focused on your goals.

Don't feel guilty. Guilt is a wasted emotion. When we say yes to too much, we're saying no to ourselves for something else. Think it through before you commit to anything. We all want to do our best to pitch in, but does that request to watch the neighbor's kids mean you're not cooking tonight and you lose a day from your ten-day meal plan? You may *feel* guilty, but don't *be* guilty. Acknowledge your feelings (it's okay to have them!), give them a love tap, and move on. If you don't learn how to discern when to say no, you risk losing your focus, and you will inch backward rather than forward from your goals.

Make sure your bucket has a bottom. When we fill a bucket with everything we need to take care of ourselves, we are in a better position to help others. Your bucket needs to have a bottom on it so you know how much you can put in. Make sure there's plenty of room for taking care of yourself, having fun, and planning your plate with amazing unprocessed meals every day!

Change your habits to change your routine. Anything you spend time on becomes a routine. If you're scrolling social media and getting distracted by requests that don't align with your vision, that

(Continues)

18

(Learn To Powerfully Say No Continued)

will become your routine, and it will be harder to accomplish your goals. But when you start putting what you want your day to look like into your daily routine, that changes everything. Think of the person you want to become. Consider your role models. What is the best version of yourself? Imagine yourself there and picture what your ideal day would look like. When does your day start? What are you doing first thing? What are you eating? Who are you with? What do you look like? How do you feel? What do you want to accomplish? What can you shift out so you have more time to cook healthy meals for yourself? Write it out, establish a routine based on what you've discovered, and schedule it on your calendar. What are you going to give up so you can find time for what you really want in your life?

Step 2

Make a Decision

When people tell me, "I've tried everything and nothing works, so I guess I'll try this," I know that the Transformation Triangle won't be their magic bullet. That's because they haven't truly decided. The big decisions in life—such as getting married, having kids, and getting off the couch and taking charge, really taking charge of your health—don't just happen. The commonality in everyone I've successfully worked with—including myself—is deciding that change is possible. What comes first is not the action but the *decision*. Decide that you are ready to commit to a healthier lifestyle and it becomes possible. That validation will open doors for you. All successful people know that to achieve their goals, they have to first make an active decision that it's possible. As soon as that client tells me, "I'm ready to do this. I am making this happen," her decision has been made. Deciding is very different from "thinking about," "considering," or "giving something a try." Deciding is a commitment.

Find supporting evidence to feed fuel to your decision and kill your self-imposed stops. If you're fifty and you don't think change is possible, recognize that is a self-imposed stop that *you* created, stop comparing yourself to twenty-somethings, and find other fifty-year-olds who are doing what you want to do. Decide that you're not too old!

As soon as you tell yourself that failure is not an option, following through comes naturally. Go all in 100 percent of the time, like an athlete who's training to win. Act as if you're already there and start doing everything it takes. You can get others to validate your excuses, but that will never change the results. Decide first, and then your dreams can become a reality. Are you ready to do this?

Exercise:
Turn Your Decision into a Declaration

Write down your name, today's date, and what you are deciding for yourself. Make it a statement. It's not a possibility—it's a commitment. No excuses allowed!

My name is _____.

On _____ I have decided that I am ready to step

into my vision of _____.

I am committed to powerfully saying NO to these things:

_____

and saying YES to: _____.

Here's my own personal declaration to get you started:

My name is Natalie Jill. As of this day, I have decided that I am going to be a strong, healthy, pain-free forty-seven-year-old woman. I am committed to powerfully saying no to things that no longer align with my vision, such as validating my excuses for pain. My disc rupture and the effects of the surgery will not define my life. I am committed to doing whatever it takes to properly rehab my body, feed it with the best nutrients and anti-inflammatory foods, and ask for help when needed. I have decided that I will not give up. I will find a solution and move without pain and get in even better shape than I was in before. I will powerfully say yes to any action that helps me remain confident and focused on my vision.

Step 3

Break Through Self-Imposed Stops

When we listen to what other people tell us, we start believing it. Self-imposed stops, or limiting beliefs, are a major mind-set roadblock, and the same goes for negative self-talk. Too set in your ways? Too out of shape? Any time you put *too* in front of a word, you're putting a cap on your dreams. Self-imposed stops give us a false sense of protection and comfort, like a security blanket with holes in it. Self-imposed stops can even have the potential to destroy your career. Before I created the Transformation Triangle, the self-imposed stop of *I'm too old* almost ended mine. Stop stopping yourself!

Losing your self-imposed stops is your secret weapon to achieving your goals. How often do you hear yourself bringing up a reason or excuse for why you can't do something, such as "Why bother, because it never works out" or "It's too late for me to change"? If you don't hear it from yourself, it might come from friends or family members or social media. A self-imposed stop is *not* a fact; it's just something you tell yourself. But it *is* true that it acts as a barrier to your reaching your goals and shuts off your options.

What do self-imposed stops cost you?

1. **They let you stay comfortable.** You don't have to take action because you have a good reason *not* to.

2. **They lower your hopes and dreams, if they don't kill them.** You tell yourself you can't, so you won't. If you tell yourself you can't go for that promotion or give up junk food, you're killing the option of it ever happening.

3. **They increase procrastination.** Since you haven't met your goals yet, you aren't motivated to start, which creates a vicious cycle of procrastination.

4. **They allow you to validate your excuses.** "Excuses or solutions, you decide" is a slogan I've been using since I started Natalie Jill Fitness. We all have excuses, but we also have a choice. You can try to validate your excuses and find evidence to back you up from friends and family. But nothing ever changes with that kind of negative "support."

As long as we continue to believe our self-imposed stops, we can't change. We can't break through that glass ceiling. If you tell yourself you don't like to exercise, it will get harder and harder to work out and you'll never reach your workout goals. Even I have been guilty of that self-imposed stop. I would go to Pilates class every week, and even though I know it's great for my core, I would hate it. One day my husband, Brooks, asked me, "What would it look like if you didn't hate Pilates?" Brooks caught my self-imposed stop! Because of that shift in perspective, I loved Pilates that day.

How to Get Past Self-Imposed Stops

1. **Identify what they are.** What comes up for you repeatedly that keeps you from going for your dreams and goals?

2. **Write them down.** Every time your mind engages in a self-imposed stop, write it down and turn it around. "I'm too busy" becomes "I'm making time to get things done." "I'm too fat and lazy" becomes "I'm getting stronger." "I'm not worthy" becomes "I'm working on being my best me." Pay attention to what you believe is true about yourself. As my cousin Liana says, "Check yourself before you wreck yourself."

3. **Figure out why you believe your self-imposed stops are true.** Where did they originate? Who told you that you weren't smart or capable? What was that first memory? Go deep.

4. **Think about the opposite reality.** If the opposite were true, what would that look like and feel like? What would you do differently? If your house is a chaotic mess, ask yourself what it would look like if you weren't constantly in a state of overwhelm. How would it be if you came home to a superorganized house? Imagine feeling calm, relaxed, and peaceful and being more present with your family. If you can't visualize what is possible, you don't give yourself that possibility.

5. **Ask yourself what you would have to do to bring that reality to life.** What would you have to do differently to make it happen? How would you have to shift your day? Look from the perspective of your vision, not your self-imposed stop.

6. **Stop attaching your identity to your self-imposed stop.** For example, my grandparents had cancer, and many people in my family have had type 2 diabetes and heart disease. My dad died at age forty-nine of a heart attack. But there's no way I'm going to fall into the mind-set of thinking I'm genetically doomed. When I had emergency back surgery, my self-imposed stops went through the roof. But I stopped those stops by making dietary shifts, getting serious about physical therapy, and making some adjustments to my workouts.

7. **Take actions to prove it's wrong.** If you've heard that weight gain, mood swings, and memory loss go hand in hand with changing hormones, learn how to take your unprocessed lifestyle up a notch with my ten-day meal plan (page 158) and changes to your fitness routine (page 257). Then, check in and see if those changes really are inevitable.

Breaking through self-imposed stops is the missing link for many of my clients: once accomplished, everything starts to shift. What self-imposed stops have gotten in the way of you achieving your dreams?

HOW SARAH LOST HER SELF-IMPOSED STOPS

Sarah was in her forties and extremely overweight when she came to me, and she had been carrying that extra weight for a long time. She told me that nothing worked for her, that being overweight was just part of who she was. She kept trying new workout programs and diets, but what she failed to see was that enormous self-imposed stop hanging over her head. Sarah's self-imposed stop was "I am genetically predisposed to being overweight."

I explained to Sarah that she didn't need to give up more food groups or further restrict what she ate. She still had to work the Transformation Triangle—and she did—but her biggest job would be to lose that self-imposed stop. She had to replace it with a belief that losing weight was possible for her. She did, and if you were to look at Sarah now, she is so lean that people actually think that she is genetically *blessed!*

Exercise:
Turn Around Your Self-Imposed Stops

Think about your self-imposed stops and pick one that you'd like to work with today. Close your eyes and change the story in your mind. What would that look like? What does it feel like? What if it were different? How can you turn it around? Rephrase your self-imposed stop and turn it into a new *what if* statement.

Self-imposed stop: _____

What if: _____

For example, the self-imposed stop "I am too tired" becomes "I am an energy magnet. I eat and stay hydrated for optimal focus and energy, and I avoid people, places, and foods that suck energy away from me."

Step 4

Find Your Driving Core Motivator

Your driving core motivator, or DCM, is your "why," taken a few steps deeper. It's the real, soul-searching reason you want to make change. It's why you get up every day, and it's what makes all the work you do to get there worth it. You can go ten levels deep to get at your why, but your DCM will be found as the feeling *behind* that why. Once you've found your DCM, declare it. Let it *become* you. It's what's going to define how you act in the world as you work your way toward realizing your goals.

Your DCM is something bigger than you. Maybe you want to reclaim your energy. You want to get out of bed without dreading getting dressed. You want to be out of pain. Or you want to be a role model to your kids. Your DCM is usually connected to something you really care about. It will change depending on where you are at in your life and what your current goals are. Mine has changed many times throughout my life.

My first DCM emerged more than twenty years ago when I lost my father. I was very close to my dad. He was my everything, my sense of worth in the world, and he was the person I went to for approval and validation. When he died of a heart attack at the young age of forty-nine, it shook my world. He didn't smoke or drink, and he wasn't overweight. How could someone so healthy just die? But when I learned about hidden factors, such as clogged arteries and visceral fat (fat around the organs), I got a different perspective on fitness, diet, and health. People might have thought I was working out because I wanted to look and feel a certain way. Of course, that was true, but my DCM became deep health and not repeating my dad's cycle.

Years later, after having my daughter, I went through a divorce. I fell into a depression, gained weight, and felt stuck. Just telling myself I should lose weight wasn't enough to motivate me. But I wanted to have energy to play with my daughter, watch her grow up, and give her the confidence to be her best self. I wanted to be the healthiest role model for her possible. And I didn't want her to go through the same type of loss that I experienced. That was when being there for my daughter became my DCM. Focusing on my daughter as my DCM is what has allowed me to keep going for the past decade. Deciding to lose the fat allowed me to gain energy and increase my self-esteem. I had a new passion, which led me to build a business and a new career helping people.

Through that new career, I've added someone else to my DCM: *you*. If I don't eat an unprocessed diet and stay in shape, I let you down. I need to look, feel, and *be* the part so I can stay true to my words. My motivation is to motivate you to find your DCM and realize your goals!

Now is the time to dig deep. So many of us want to feel better, but is the way we are currently feeling serving a purpose? What would it take to take your health back? What would happen if you realized all your goals? What is holding you back? Get curious, like a child, and ask yourself lots of questions. What really drives you? That is your DCM.

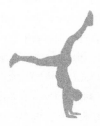

Exercise:
Find Your Driving Core Motivator

Take the time, space, and focus to identify your why. Then, go several levels deeper to reach your DCM.

For example:

How do you want to feel?

I want to get my energy back and feel motivated.

Why is having energy and feeling motivated important?

Because I want to be social and have fun again and be excited about my day.

Why is that important to you?

Because right now I feel lonely and sad.

What happens then?

I get depressed and isolated.

There it is: The DCM is *I want to feel connected.*

This exercise can be applied to any goal or vision you have, whether it's a personal goal or a physical one. Only when you get to your DCM will you see long-lasting change. It may take some time, but stay with it.

Step 5

Don't Just Try—Commit!

What if I told you to *try* to pick up a pencil? The pencil doesn't budge. Trying won't get you that pencil—you just have to bend over and grab it! Likewise, if you just think about something, it doesn't usually happen.

Make a commitment to whatever you set out to do in life. Dedication follows, and results come easily. When you understand the distinction between trying and committing, nothing will stand in your way. When you try something, it doesn't mean it's going to happen. When you commit to something, you do it. There's no chance to back out of it. Think about all the times you succeeded at what you set out to accomplish. Chances are you went further than trying—you really stuck to your guns and committed.

I'd like to ask you to commit to not using the word *try* anymore, because that word is giving you an out. People tell me they're going to *try* to look for a new job, *try* to save money this year, or *try* to lose weight. But what inevitably happens is something else becomes a priority and the intention is lost. But when you commit to something, that becomes your priority—you stick to it and make it happen.

When I decided to leave corporate America, I never said I was going to *try* to start a health and fitness business. I committed to it. Even though there were some ups and downs, because I had made the commitment, backing out wasn't an option. Think of it this way: When you know 100 percent that something is going to work, you're going to do it. If you don't think it's going to work, you'll prove that it won't. Don't leave room for doubt and your goals will become reality.

And once you commit to your goals, work backward.

First think fantasy goals: *If anything was possible, what would that look like?*

Then, for the long term: *What would be possible in five years?*

And for the short term: *What could be possible in a year?*

Finally, daily: *What would I need to do every day for those short-term goals to become reality?*

Exercise:
Stop Trying and Commit!

What have you been trying to do? List everything that comes to mind. What are you willing to turn into a commitment? Choose one thing you can commit to and turn this into a statement for yourself; for example, "I'm committing to putting myself first and taking the weight off" or "I'm committed to creating a happier life for myself." Put it in your journal or on a Post-it and stick it to your bathroom mirror.

Step 6

Add the Good

Are the people around you a positive force, or do they breed negativity? Are friends and family bettering themselves and want the same for you? What are you feeding your brain? Is it useful information, such as from books, podcasts, and blogs that support your goals? Or are you watching reality TV and gossip shows that make you feel bad about yourself? Is social media encouraging or a waste of time? Are you following yet another diet plan without learning about true nourishment?

Your inner circle and others you surround yourself with can be your daily dose of good or can derail you from your goals. We've all heard the expression "You're the sum of those you surround yourself with." When it comes to nutrition, who you surround yourself with is critical. If you are on a healthy eating track and everyone else around you is trying to derail you, it wouldn't be a surprise if you started to doubt yourself. People have told me that if they had the kind of support that I have in my life, they could get their health back or lose the extra fat. My response is always the same: "I made a choice." I took a chance and looked for people to support me. I made a decision and created my reality.

Consider doing a social media cleanse: unfriend and unfollow anyone who doesn't make you feel happy, empowered, inspired, motivated, and encouraged to work toward your goals. Don't give them a place in your space. That will give you bonus time in your life to add in the good.

How do you know who are the right people for you? Here's what I do: I keep a list on my phone of everyone in my world who makes me feel motivated, energized, and happy when I'm around them. I call them my power people, people who help me become a better person. If you don't have this in your life, you can find inspiration by following your passion through podcasts, social media, books, or classes. Become a student from afar. There's always room to add more positivity to your life.

I think of my life as a bus. Who inspires and motivates you in your life? Positive people, healthy food, movement, and encouraging words all get a seat on my bus, and I pick them up daily. As you let in more of the good, there's less room for those who drain you or are taking their life in a different direction. And there's less room for junk food, lack of motivation, and self-imposed stops. You've got to let them off the bus. Instead of thinking of all the things you *can't* do today, turn it around and ask yourself who and what you can pick up and put on your bus, then make realizing your goals your destination!

Exercise:
How Much Goodness Can You Add to Your Day?

In the following space, list twenty good things you can add to your day and choose one every day for twenty days. Then see what happens. Some examples of what you might list could include "playing with my dog," "moving my body," "connecting with a friend," "listening to a podcast," "eating a healthy snack," "going for a walk outside," or "reading a few chapters from an uplifting book."

Goodness I Can Add to My Day

1. _____
2. _____
3. _____
4. _____
5. _____
6. _____
7. _____
8. _____
9. _____
10. _____
11. _____
12. _____
13. _____
14. _____
15. _____
16. _____
17. _____
18. _____
19. _____
20. _____

Step 7

Create a Morning Routine

We all wake up with our to-do lists, the things we don't like about ourselves, what he said or she said, and so on. Then, the next thing we do is start scrolling social media on our phone (sound familiar?). Well, I took a radical step and put my phone in another room when I go to bed! Now, the first thing I do is literally dump out what's in my brain (see the following exercise). I put it out and throw it out without acting it out!

After the Brain Dump, I make a quick gratitude list on a notepad or journal with three things I'm grateful for. It can be anything, from my comfy sheets to the fact that I have access to clean water and can move. Then, I set an intention for the day: "I'm going to be peaceful today" or "I'm going to have a productive day" or "I'm going to be early to my appointments today."

Then, as I'm getting dressed and making a healthy breakfast (don't skip that step—it's important to fuel yourself with lots of good nutrition in the morning), I get into learning mode. I listen to an audiobook or podcast so I can take in information before I check in with what other people need of me. You can listen to whatever nourishes your brain and soul, be it Scripture, a motivational talk, or the latest in your field to keep you at the top of your game.

After taking in info, I create a must-do list for the day. It's not a list of twenty things I need to get done. Rather, it's three things that I *get* to do. If your goal is better well-being and more fat loss, think of three things that will move you toward those goals; for example, "I'm going to go for a walk. I'm going to yoga. I'm going to get my lunches ready for the week." Find time for those must-dos in your schedule before letting the day take over.

What does your ideal morning look like? Which habits do you want to keep, and which would you like to change? What do you need to do to create a morning routine?

Exercise:
The Daily Brain Dump

1. Have a pen and piece of paper (not your journal) handy at your bedside when you go to sleep.

2. When you first wake up, rather than reach for your phone, grab your paper and pen and write down any and everything that comes into your mind, from the good, to the ugly, to the indifferent. Don't be shy! The Brain Dump is for your eyes only.

3. Toss it!

There's something supercleansing about writing it all down and throwing it out. It gives a fresh, new start to your morning. Now instead of carrying all that around or venting to friends or coworkers, you can be an inspiration to them. After the Brain Dump, your brain will be clear and ready to take in new information.

Note that your Brain Dump is for your eyes only. If anything action-oriented comes out of it, put it on your must-do list, but dump everything else out.

Step 8

Create a Focus Flow

You get what you're looking for. That may sound simplistic, but we tend to look for evidence for whatever we believe or whatever we're doing. If your focus is on weight you've gained, you'll look around for other people who've gained weight for validation. If you believe that you're too old to get in shape, you will continue to find evidence to support that. If I listened to my friends and popular media, I would never have entered into launching a fitness and nutrition business in my late thirties. I had to believe it for myself and find role models who supported my vision. If you focus on connecting with people your age or older who are accomplishing what you want to accomplish, you start shifting in that direction.

Another way we find supporting evidence is to look at others to validate our excuses. Validating your excuses will *never* help you break through them, nor is enrolling others in validating your excuses.

What you focus on expands. If you think positive thoughts, you will attract positivity. If you focus on the negative, you'll attract more negativity. That's the law of attraction in full effect. Remember *The Little Engine That Could*? The law of attraction is like that. Once you really decide to do something, I promise you will find evidence to keep you headed in the right direction!

WHAT STRESS DOES TO OUR BODY

Whereas some short-term stressors might make us lose our appetite, chronic stress over the long haul can actually cause us to *gain* weight.

Long-term chronic stress makes us want to eat more, and more of the wrong foods. Say your boss suddenly dumps a project on you just as you were about to leave for the weekend. Or maybe she wasn't happy with a job you put a ton of effort into. While you're dealing with life's daily stresses, you see a vending machine and all of a sudden that candy starts calling your name. That's your primitive brain engaging the fight-or-flight reaction. Your brain doesn't know the difference between dealing with your boss and running from a tiger. Same thing if you are going through a divorce or dealing with a sick parent or a cranky coworker. Your body is wired to think it *needs* the extra calories to deal with a life-threatening situation.

Whenever we're stressed, levels of the stress hormone cortisol start to rise very quickly. Increased stress levels lead to increased insulin levels, and our blood sugar typically starts to drop. To self-regulate, our body starts to crave sugary and starchy foods because it wants to get us back to normal. That's how the term *comfort foods* came about. The more stress we have, the more cortisol our body produces, the more we want to eat comfort foods, and the more weight we gain. What's even worse is that long-term elevated levels of cortisol elevate our blood pressure and are directly implicated in belly fat.

Stress can also affect our metabolism. We are wired to digest our food stress-free and relaxed and to take care of our nervous system first. We can be eating a healthy diet, but if we're in a state of stress, our digestion won't be up to speed. We won't absorb all the nutrients and our metabolism loses ground, and we pack on pounds even though we are doing everything right with our diet. And this state of affairs becomes even more pronounced as we get older and our hormones start to shift.

The first step to calming stress is recognizing that stress is there. Then, add mindful, calming practices to your life. Here are a few to get you started:

Meditate. If you just rolled your eyes here, see page 39.

Take a walk. Leave your cell phone at home and get in touch with your environment. Notice sights, sounds, and smells. If you take your dog for a walk, notice her curiosity. How does your body feel as it's moving? How does the air feel on your face? Distance yourself from your to-dos by being fully present on your walk.

Read. Get lost in a good book and start shifting your focus. If you have trouble diving in, try playing some soothing background music, grabbing a cup of tea, and creating a special space to read in. In my home I have a room set up with a comfy chair, candles, relaxing paintings on the wall, and a cozy blanket. I know when I go in there, I will be in reading mode, and it instantly relaxes me.

Take up a hobby or craft. Cooking is a fun one, especially with all the delicious healthy recipes you'll be learning!

Listen to music. Music truly alters your state. For relaxation, I love listening to Enigma, Enya, and Cirque du Soleil songs. For energy and creativity, I turn to show tunes. I enjoy listening to the soundtrack from *The Greatest Showman*. Don't be afraid to sing along, and loudly! If you use a music app, such as iTunes, you can see the lyrics right on your phone. I have been known to really belt it out . . . you are lucky you haven't heard me, as I am not exactly a talented singer, but it truly works for stress reduction!

Pray. Regardless of your religious preference or beliefs, praying or focusing on a higher power can help you focus out and surrender.

Do nothing. Literally. Remember the days of flying before we had laptops, cell phones, and iPads? I'd stare out into the clouds from the airplane, just daydreaming. Where did those days go? Bring them back! Do nothing and allow your mind to wander and dream.

Get a massage. Be truly present and speak up if you need to make any adjustments, so as to have a fully enjoyable experience.

Exercise:
Attract a New Reality

Envision a new reality. Note it in the following space (or in your journal or a Post-it note that you can stick to your bathroom mirror). Commit to it, and watch how you start attracting evidence to support that new belief!

My new reality:

_____

_____

_____

_____

_____

_____

_____

_____

_____

_____

_____

_____

_____

_____

_____

_____

MY VERSION OF MEDITATION

Maybe you're not into meditation, but you know it's good for you. I hear you! But what to do with your racing mind and never-ending thoughts? When my head starts spinning with a million ideas, to-dos, and the stress of the day, my natural tendency is to go into control mode. If I feel like I can get it under control, delegate it, or micromanage it so I can check things off the list, the stress will go away. Of course, this never works for long. It always comes back when more is added to my plate. Trying to control it costs me greatly. It makes me less than present and not fun to be around.

So, when I'm in that place, this is what I do to calm down and de-stress. I focus on four words: *patient, present, playful,* and *loving.* These words are my authentic self—the real me before the stress. Now, if you were to meet me in stress mode, you would *not* describe me as any of those. But when I am living those words, I am fun to be around, creative, and relaxed. I become calm and focused.

For me, meditation looks like this: I put some relaxing music on my headphones, I sit with my eyes closed, I focus on my breath, and I repeat those four words. I say them over and over to myself: *patient, present, playful,* and *loving.* I take a survey of my body and I direct my breath to where I feel tension. At first my head spins, I panic, and I try to control the experience, and then I let myself sink into it and patient, present, playful, loving Natalie comes back.

What are your four words? First, think of ways that are *not* serving you and come up with words that express the opposite. For example, if you are frequently rigid or strict, *free* could be your word. If you are always controlled, *easygoing* could be your word. When you've picked your four words, breathe deeply and repeat them to yourself. You can do this anytime, even for a few seconds or a minute, to bring a peaceful presence to your day.

Step 9

Create New Habits

How to create new habits? First, establish which current habits aren't serving you well and notice the emotion that's connected with them. To quit a habit, you've got to replace it with something that satisfies. I used to eat late at night, and often the wrong foods (can you relate?). To shift out of that habit, after I finished dinner, I would brush my teeth. Brushing my teeth now marks the end of eating for the day.

Another late-night habit I used to have was checking my cell phone. And then, I'd check it again first thing in the morning. I was wasting all sorts of time on social media. So, what I decided to do was set my alarm and put my cell phone in a different room when I went to bed. Now when I climb into bed at night, I can't reach my phone, so I go to sleep earlier. When the alarm sounds in the morning, I have to get up and go into the other room to turn it off. Once I'm out of my warm, cozy bed, instead of checking social media, I do the Daily Brain Dump (see page 34) and I'm up and ready to start my day in a productive way.

Another way to create new habits is to minimize your options. The more options we have, the harder it is to stick to goals. Think of it as a buffet at a restaurant. When there are endless choices, you're more likely to pile on the food. If you minimize your options, you're more likely to eat just the right amount.

Exercise:
Choose Habits to Commit To

What are three habits that are sabotaging your path to health?
What are the healthy habits you will choose?

For example: Checking your phone and scrolling before your morning routine leaves your morning to chance. What you find on social media, e-mail, or texts can affect your mind-set for the rest of the day. It can even cause you to get you off track and ditch your routine altogether. Instead, pick a mindful, productive way to start your day. For instance, work on a gratitude list, meditate, listen to a podcast, or read from an inspiring book first. Eat a healthy breakfast and get some exercise before you start to scroll.

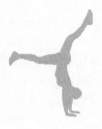

Step 10

Connect with the Right People

Connecting with others not only makes us happier, it makes us healthier, more mentally fit, and apt to live a longer life. Tending to your relationships, being accountable to the people in your life, can be just as important as eating the right foods and taking impeccable care of your body. As the saying goes, birds of a feather flock together. Finding a person, people, or group who are on the same path as you means everything.

Make a declaration and publicly share your intention so you can keep your focus and be accountable to others and yourself.

Join an accountability group to connect with people on the same path or find a friend who will commit to checking in with you at a certain time each week to make sure you both follow through.

Connection is a cure for much of what troubles us. One of the side effects of the digital age is that there's less face time, more of a focus in than out. When we connect with people, it brings us happy energy and makes us feel alive again. And it makes us accountable. Successful people are accountable for their own successes and failures regardless of the circumstances. They take responsibility. They do not blame others or hunt for excuses but connect with others so they can follow through.

When I meet positive, goal-oriented, successful, happy, and energetic people, I want to know more about them, and if we have a connection, I want them in my life. I find ways to be around them so I can be accountable to them. Consider yourself the sum of the people you surround yourself with.

Many of the women who come to work with me have been depressed and withdrawn because of excess weight and health issues that have come with age. When we feel bad about ourselves, we tend to become isolated. When we think things are happening *to* us, rather than *for* us, we feel like a victim. And when we feel like a victim, we're giving up hope for change because we lose responsibility and accountability. But when we connect with others, it opens up and energizes us. The more responsibility we take, the more in power we feel. Connecting with others in similar circumstances and working toward improving together makes a big difference. Who in your life inspires you? Makes a list. Then, pick someone from that list and tell that person about your goal. Ask him or her to help you be accountable and to call you out if you don't follow through.

Accept accountability for everything that happens in your life, from success to failure. As soon as you blame something on someone else, you can't control it. But when you're accountable, you can transform it. Sure, there will always be people we can blame. Everyone has a past and a story. Recognize that and move on. Take control of your future. It's amazing what happens when you share your vision and become accountable. Your vision comes to life!

Exercise:
It's Nobody Else's Fault

Write down this statement: "It is nobody else's fault." Make it big. Make it bold. Put it somewhere you'll see it. Be accountable to yourself and create the future you envision. If we continue to blame others for our circumstances, we don't allow ourselves the power to create change. The sooner we accept accountability and recognize our role, the sooner we are able to break through and make changes.

10 WAYS TO HAPPINESS DAILY

It's easy to let our daily lives consume us. We let people get to us. We allow others to determine our moods. Maybe you work around people who literally drain you. Maybe your kids are away and you miss them. And even if you're generally happy-go-lucky, it never hurts to add a little more sunshine to your day! Here are ten simple actions you can take that will make a huge change in the way you feel, and they require no more than a few minutes out of your day. I promise they'll make you more productive, too, giving greater value to the time you spend on *you*.

1. **Smile.** Try this experiment for a day: Make eye contact and smile (even if it is forced) with as many people as you can. You'll be amazed at how much better you feel. Smiling scientifically tricks your mind into thinking you are happy and releases those feel-good chemicals known as endorphins.

2. **Play more.** Be your authentic self. What would the kid in you do? Have a good laugh. Laughing is not only good for the soul, it's great for your abs (really! Remember the last time you laughed so hard your belly hurt?). Don't be afraid to get a little goofy. Need help? Your computer or phone will give you endless opportunities for a good belly laugh; just don't let yourself get diverted for more than a couple of minutes.

3. **Accept you are worthy and practice self-love.** Be your biggest fan. Look in the mirror and tell yourself at least five things you love about yourself. It can be something physical or a personality trait—it makes no difference. What matters is that you remember why you're awesome and genuinely believe it. Positive affirmations are

important not only to our happiness but to our success in meeting our goals.

4. **Inspire yourself.** Where do you get your inspiration from? I can promise you that comparing yourself to others won't get you to your happy place. Spend a few minutes listening to your favorite music, drawing, or writing in your journal.

5. **Connect.** Call a friend or family member and catch up. We get so consumed by the day to day that we forget how important the little things are. It is important to stay sincerely connected to the ones we love. So, get up from behind that keypad, avoid the temptation to text, and pick up the phone.

6. **Be grateful.** Do more, get more, be more . . . with all that striving, sometimes we can forget how much we already have. Take a moment, close your eyes, and be grateful for all there is in your life. Do you have a roof over your head? Do you have a door that closes? There are so many people in the world who can't even say yes to that. It's the small things we take for granted. Be appreciative of all that you have.

7. **Accept and shift.** Accept the things that cannot change, then think about what you *can* change. What is one thing you're unhappy with? Take one step—even if it's just thinking about it—in the direction of shifting it right now.

8. **Live in the present.** Let just now be your focus. Let *you* be your focus. Not what he or she is doing, said, or has . . . just you. It's never too late to start loving yourself and making this world a better place. We are all in this this together!

(Continues)

(10 Ways to Happiness Daily Continued)

9. **Eat a nutrient-rich, healing snack.** Eating clean makes you feel better from the inside out. When you feel lazy and lethargic and eat a starchy or sugary comfort food, you inevitably feel even *more* lethargic and unmotivated. Instead, treat your body to a healthy snack and see what a difference it makes in your mood.

10. **Move your body.** We've all heard of the term *runner's high*. Exercising releases endorphins that reduce your perception of pain, be it physical or mental. It has been proven that releasing endorphins through exercise can reduce stress, lower anxiety and depression, improve sleep, and increase self-esteem. And exercising is even more important as our hormones start to shift. Pick one of the moves from pages 259 to 273, walk or run around the block, do some yoga sequences, or get up and dance. Take a few minutes out to move!

You've made a commitment to affect change in your life. Don't underestimate the power you have inside you. You're starting to see results already because you've set goals and *feel* you're already there. You're remembering to smile, play, and bring in the good whenever you can. You can see the path before you with insight and clarity. The next step is to connect mind and body by nourishing yourself with the healthiest food on earth so you can truly start aging in reverse!

Transformation

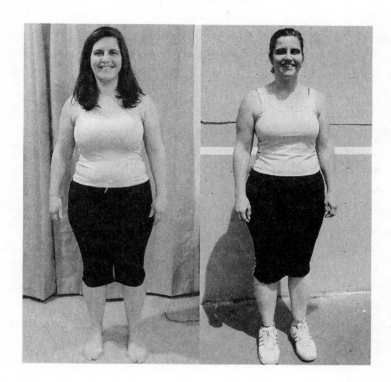

MIRA

"I Stopped Putting Everyone Else First and Put Myself First"

When I first came across Natalie Jill, I was intrigued by her work with mind-set. On one of her videos, she explained that you could get anyone to lose weight, but if you don't switch your mind-set, it won't stick. It seemed like a different way of approaching weight loss, and I wanted to know more. Part of my research as a scientist at a software company involves getting people to learn new things. So, what I found interesting about Natalie's work is how she homes in on the motivation part of getting fit.

The previous year had been stressful. I have two kids, and my daughter had just turned two. I had gained 15 pounds and was suffering from back pain. My body was out of whack, and I felt I needed a change.

I started by homing in on my vision. My vision was to be confident, fun, light, and creative. Confident in work, fun in spirit, light in weight and carefree, and creative to balance my work in science. My job is nine to five, but then I'd come home, have dinner with my family, and jump back on the computer. Natalie taught me about the importance of carving out time in my day for myself so my vision could become a reality.

Culturally, I was taught that women take care of the family, so I uncovered that my self-imposed stop was that others always come first. Every day there's someone to take care of at home and at work, and every moment there's something to do. When I started journaling, I came to understand that for me to be really great at what I do, I have to take care of myself. If I'm not happy or healthy, I can't take care of others at my best. I learned that it was possible to do everything and still make time for myself. I started out by taking a walk after dinner, time that was just for me. Then, I got back into tennis, and I'm now playing regularly. There's nothing better than getting in that perfect stroke! Working out has become a habit, and days when I skip I feel like I'm missing something.

My mother and grandmother all got chubby as they aged, so I thought it was inevitable that I eventually would be round. I thought my genetics were just what they were and there was nothing I could do about it. But after learning that Natalie Jill became a fitness model in her forties and remembering that some of my friends who were heavier younger lost a huge amount of weight, I reversed that self-imposed stop. I didn't have to be the person I thought I had to be.

Since I started the Aging in Reverse program, I am in a much better place. I have always eaten minimal processed foods and lots of vegetables. With Aging in Reverse, I have really upped the vegetables, and if I don't eat enough of them now, I crave them. The recipes are easy and really amazing. I rely on the protein balls, fudge, crackers, and pesto, which I add to everything. In the past, I'd pick and choose from plans, but this was the first time I followed a plan exactly. I lost 2½ pounds in the ten days. Normally I lose a pound a week, so for me that was quite a change, and I was really happy with that kind of sustainable weight loss. And most of all, I've gotten myself back. Instead of putting everyone else first, I've learned to put myself first!

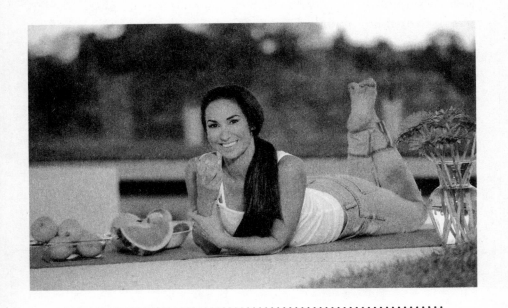

Once we get in touch with our body and eliminate the foods that are harming us . . . an amazing thing happens. We start to crave and eat the right things, and we feel truly nourished. It's like finding the fountain of youth!

PART 2

Plan Your Plate

Maybe you believe you've been eating really well and doing everything right, but suddenly you put on weight around your midsection or are feeling bloated much of the time. Perhaps you're sluggish, having trouble focusing, or even suffering from aches and pains, the telltale signs of inflammation. While an entire industry of solutions has sprung up to help us feel lean and mean as we age, don't overlook one of the most simple and effective weapons. That, of course, is the food we eat. Food is the most powerful medicine we have.

Once we get in touch with our body and eliminate the foods that are harming us—and this may include foods that until just recently served us—an amazing thing happens. We start to crave and eat the right things, and we feel truly nourished. It's like finding the fountain of youth!

This part of the book will teach you exactly how to plan your plate in a way that directly impacts both the way you feel and your fat loss. This is the time for finding optimal nutrition. Avoiding certain foods and reaching for others is even more important now than ever. It's time to stop guessing what to eat and learn how to give your body exactly what it needs to thrive. Instead of mindlessly following another diet plan or program, it's time to learn which foods are inflammatory and how to avoid them as well as which foods are most nourishing for you. This ties back to our vision from the beginning of the book: after you've changed your state, it will no longer be a struggle to plan your plate. You've tackled the tip of the Transformation Triangle. You've honed in on your vision, you've found your driving core motivator, and you're committed to making changes to meet your body where it is. Let's get started!

Step 1

Create a New Jump Start

On pages 1 to 6, I shared the story of my recent health issues. In my determination to bypass pain's warning signs, push through it, and act as if my body was exactly the same as it was ten years before, I almost did permanent damage to myself. From that humbling experience, I looked into what was no longer working for me and I set out to understand the link between inflammation and pain. I needed a new jump start to reset my body. I had to plan my plate differently. I found that when I drastically reduced or removed several potential inflammation triggers—grains (in addition to the gluten I gave up when I was diagnosed with celiac disease), dairy, legumes (including soy), and processed corn—from my daily meals, my pain decreased dramatically. Honing in on what worked and didn't work for me became my mission. That mission also included volumizing my veggies, including more fermented foods in my diet, and challenging myself to eat from ten groups of superfoods every day.

Put an End to Calorie Counting

Counting calories and cutting fat aren't part of planning your plate (go ahead and do a happy dance!). In case you were wondering, calories aren't those little things that sneak into your closet at night and change the size of your clothes. Calories are a measure of energy, and they're what determine whether

THE MISSING LINK

Hey there, I see you! If in your eagerness to take unprocessed up a notch, you skipped over the first section of the book, Change Your State (pages 11 to 49), stop right there! This plan will not get you the radical lasting results that I know it can if you don't work with all three parts. I encourage you to back up before jumping in. Changing your state has to happen before *anything* else happens. If you simply follow a new lifestyle plan without engaging your mind-set, you'll inevitably lose motivation and won't achieve the results you were hoping for. Once you understand the importance of mind-set, you can use the skills you've learned to listen to your body and feed it what it truly needs. Changing your state is that missing link that makes *everything* possible.

we lose or gain fat. In black-and-white simplified terms, 1 pound of weight is equal to 3,500 calories. So, if you want to lose 1 pound of fat, you would essentially need to create a calorie deficit of 3,500 calories, or 500 calories a day for a week, either through eating less or exercising more. But nothing ever really is black and white, and relying strictly on calorie counting is not the magic bullet to lasting fat-loss success. Eating 500 calories of jelly beans is not going to get you better results than eating 1,500 calories of fruits and vegetables. And 1,500 calories of fruits and vegetables will make you feel 100 percent different from 1,500 calories of jelly beans! Counting calories can actually be a time-consuming distraction and can work counter to your efforts. Instead, concentrate on the balance of protein, fats, and carbs on your plate. One of my followers recently posted that she tried an app to count calories and all it did was make her think about food all the time!

I'm not saying you should completely ignore calories (and yes, I've included calorie counts for my recipes, because many people find it useful to have them as a general guideline), but relying on calorie counting alone is not the way to healthy weight loss. It is impossible to accurately track calories. If you ask how many calories are in an apple, for example, the answer is elusive. There are too many questions. How big is that apple? How ripe is it? Most people drastically overestimate how many calories they burn in a day and underestimate how much they consume. This inevitably leads to failure, and I'm not up for anything that's a setup for failure! The great news is that it will be very hard to put on weight with the unprocessed foods you'll now be enjoying.

....
Transformation
....

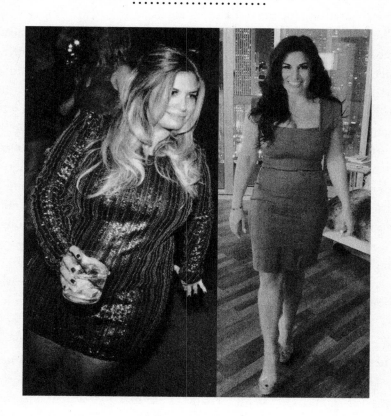

NICOLE
"I Put an End to Calorie Counting"

Before I started working Natalie's plan, I had gained more than 40 pounds in two years. I had moved to the Midwest from Southern California and was in an unhealthy relationship. I missed my friends and family, so I turned to food as a comfort.

I'm the national sales director for a tech company, and I travel a lot for work. I'm in an airport and hotel three or four times a week, and the food prep required on other diets made sticking to them next to impossible. I tried everything, from Atkins to Whole30, keto, nutrition shakes, and personal trainers, to take the weight off. I spent thousands of dollars and none of it worked. I even used an app to log my food and count calories, but I couldn't commit to anything for more than two weeks.

When I started Natalie's program, the first step I took was to clean my kitchen of anything "non–Natalie Jill"; i.e., processed foods. By unprocessing my diet, I noticed an instant change to my mood and energy. I could go all day without the extra carbs: I could find simple foods, such as hard-boiled eggs, fish, shrimp, and vegetables even at the airport, making sticking to the program easy. I loved the unlimited veggies! And I would make sure to bring nuts, fruit, and other unprocessed snacks along with me. The simplicity of the plan made me realize that I wasn't really giving up anything; rather, I was simply changing my balance. What a relief to give up calorie counting completely! For exercise, I started small by walking to work rather than taking a cab, and if I didn't have time to go to the gym, I could still do something, like hold a plank for a minute here and there. Without even trying, the weight just kept coming off.

Even though I lost the entire 40 pounds, the biggest shift for me was the emotional shift. Changing my mind-set was what did it for me. I put images of love on my vision board because I wanted to find love in my life, and I added pictures of fit girls and runners to inspire me to get to the place where I could do a 5K (which I eventually did!). Whenever I would say, "I need to lose weight," I would obsess about my weight. But when I replaced that phrase with "I am happy being fit" and "I am that goal weight already," my true self would answer back, "I can do this." I committed to never look in the mirror and say, "You're fat." That had to stop.

Now when I crave carbs, I ask myself what I'm *really* craving. I understand the difference between nourishing my body and fulfilling an emotional need. When I wonder whether I should eat a food, I go back to Natalie's question "Does it come from a mom or have a seed?" It's not like I never have the slice of pizza or other cheat food. I just don't beat myself up about it anymore and then get back on track.

When I was heavier, I slept a lot. I'd go to bed around 10:30 and wouldn't get up until 9:00. I was in my early thirties, but I felt like an old lady. Now, I wake up at 5:30 without an alarm and have unlimited energy and a newfound motivation for life. I had been aging fast, but now I am aging in reverse!

The Rundown

First, I'll go into detail on what it means to be **100 percent unprocessed**. When you're eating processed foods, such as chips or cookies, your taste buds go crazy, and it becomes almost impossible to stop. That's when you fall off track. But how often do you overeat salad, apples, or fish? Think of it as addition rather than subtraction. Instead of obsessing over what you *can't* eat, think of how much of the good you can add. I'll teach you how to plan your plate so it's **balanced in protein, fats, and carbs**. People are always looking for a magic pill. There is one, and you'll find it in nature. I'll introduce the concept of **V3: Value, Volume, Vegetables**! Your plate is **added-sugar-free**, because sugar is possibly the most inflammatory substance most people eat every day. We'll cover the dangers, including unintended weight gain, of replacing sugar with artificial sweeteners. Because dairy is mucus producing, it can contribute to or cause inflammation. For that reason, this plan goes **dairy-free**. It is also **legume-free (including soy-free), gluten-free, and grain-free**, as all of these can be difficult to digest and contribute to inflammation and bloating. For many people, eliminating them can help take off those extra pounds they thought had become permanent, especially as they get older. You'll continue to add the good with **probiotic-rich fermented foods** to increase gut health and help you absorb nutrients. Keeping **hydrated**, be it from water, bone broth, soups, or salads, is key to overall good health and sustainable fat loss. You'll develop the superpower of ageless health by eating from ten categories of delicious **anti-inflammatory superfoods** every day. With nutrient-rich ingredients, including spices, chocolate, mushrooms, and neglected veggies, such as parsley stems and strawberry tops, you'll fuel your body while keeping your budget in check.

What to Expect

How can you expect to feel from this incredible infusion of goodness? You'll start noticing a difference within the first several days—your mind will be clearer, your pants won't fit so snugly, and your cravings will diminish. If you're coming straight from a processed food diet and sedentary lifestyle (congrats on making the switch!), it may seem tough at first, but give it a few days and you're going to feel as you haven't felt in decades. That's aging in reverse in action! If you are transitioning from my 7-Day Jump Start, you'll get even faster results. If you've been eating an unprocessed diet and your results are slowing down or you feel that you've come to a standstill, this will speed them up and take you to another level.

After the full ten days, you'll start feeling focused, your bloating will be gone, your moods will even out, and you'll have newfound energy. Most people take off about 5 pounds in the first week of unprocessing their diet this way. You'll feel so good that you'll want to keep going. Keep it up for a month and the results will be so steady, you won't want to stop. This is when you're invited to make it a lifestyle with the adjustments I discuss on pages 135 to 138, once you've reached your health and weight goals.

You'll continue to lose on average 2 pounds a week. It won't always be exact—some weeks, you might lose 3 pounds; and others, it might be 1 pound. If you're someone who does weekly weigh-ins, don't be discouraged on the weeks when the scale is moving more slowly (which is one good reason you might want to skip weighing yourself altogether; see below). Knowing that this is completely normal is superimportant for staying motivated, encouraged, and on track. Remember, it's not just about weight but feeling your youngest, best possible self!

Losing 2 pounds per week is a doable, safe, and sustainable goal, because it means you're losing fat. If you're thinking that sounds too slow, think of it this way: it's more than 100 pounds in a year! When you're losing weight at a faster rate, you start to tap into water weight and muscle mass. That's why any diet out there that promises you you'll lose 20 pounds in twenty days is doomed to crash. You don't want to lose muscle mass, because the more muscle you have, the more calories you use at rest, and the leaner you are.

Having good muscle mass makes your metabolism work best. Keep it consistent, keep it healthy, and your weight loss will be sustainable.

Skip the Weekly Weigh-in

The best way of tracking progress is *not* through the scale. In fact, you might even want to pack away your scale for now. Look at your body, not the scale, to assess your progress. Take pictures of yourself, ideally in a bathing suit, and include shots from the front, back, and side. Then, take measurements around your waist, stomach, thighs, and biceps. Pictures are the best way of measuring your progress. The scale number will become much less important when you see the difference in how you look. Then, I invite you to post your Before and After on my Facebook page!

Become an Expert in Meal Planning

We'll pull together what you've learned with my ten-day meal plan, and from there you'll become an expert in planning your own breakfasts, lunches, and dinners going forward. If you don't know the why behind a new way of eating, it's hard to stick to it. I'll help you understand what happens to your body when you eat certain foods and when you make healthier choices. This will enable you to make better decisions with your daily meals going forward, you won't have to rely solely on willpower, and you'll even be able to build a meal from a restaurant menu, so you don't fall off track when you eat out. When you have the education to back you up, you'll get better at it all the time.

Write It Down

To keep track of what you're eating and how you feel after, I'll be asking you to start a food log. A food log keeps you accountable, reveals gaps, tracks highs and lows so you can connect them with what you ate, enables you to figure out which foods are causing bloat, and will get you to think twice before making unwise choices. Because keeping a food log is intricately tied to getting results, I make them mandatory for all my clients. You'll find the details on page 146.

What If You're Already Following a Diet Plan?

There are so many popular diet plans to choose from, from Whole30 to paleo and Weight Watchers, and new ones are constantly popping up. As long as your plate is balanced and unprocessed, with the exception of a vegetarian/vegan diet (see page 77 for my explanation why), most plans can easily fit into this program.

Step 2

Make 100 Percent Unprocessed
the Base of Your Plate

The term *clean eating* has been getting a lot of buzz in recent years. Clean eating means different things to different people, leaving lots of room for confusion and misinterpretation. Just eating a diet high in greens or a vegan, paleo, or keto diet doesn't necessarily mean clean. Neither does eating a fat-free or sugar-free diet. Beware of the dangers of "free" foods! They often are processed junk with artificial ingredients. And remember that eating gluten-free doesn't necessarily mean unprocessed, as many gluten-free products are filled with fake ingredients.

Real clean eating simply means eating foods that are 100 percent unprocessed. If I were to give you one rule when it comes to nutrition and achieving fat loss, it would be to unprocess your diet. Everything that follows revolves around the idea of unprocessing your diet.

What does unprocessed mean exactly? The simplest way to categorize unprocessed foods is to think of foods that once had life. Foods that grew. Foods with one ingredient in their most natural state: nuts, seeds, vegetables, fruits, meat, and fish. Compare that to a bag of chips, candies, or a frozen dinner with a confusing list of components including sugar (in its many disguises), artificial sweeteners, and unhealthy oils. Instead, look for one ingredient or a few simple ingredients. Heavily processed foods tend to be

YOU GET WHAT YOU PAY FOR

It's true that processed foods are cheaper, but when you calculate lost energy and increased medical bills, the cost to your health is going to be much higher in the long run. For example, hydrogenated oils are still found in many foods. They are a superprocessed and cheap source of fat that increase shelf life but are linked with higher risk of heart disease. Canola and vegetable oils are processed oils and can be harmful to your health as well. Nitrates have been linked to cancer but can still be found in many foods, in particular bacon. Artificial sweeteners, sugar, and, even worse, high-fructose corn syrup all create cravings, insulin spikes, and changes to our taste buds. We'll cover these unnatural ingredients later in the book, but for now know that the only people benefiting from processed foods are the manufacturers and the pharmaceutical companies that are profiting from the problems the foods are causing. Shop smart and make unprocessed your mantra!

empty in nutrition and filled with empty calories. They are not only void of key nutrients, but they also have excess sodium, artificial flavors, artificial colors, and fillers—all types of things that aren't going to help you with your fat-loss goals. Because you're not eating real food, your body keeps craving more. It's confused into thinking it's still hungry when actually it's begging you for nourishment. If you can pronounce the ingredients on the label, that's a good sign!

Grains, beans, legumes, and dairy products are minimally processed to make them fit for human consumption. They can be part of an unprocessed diet. However, they can be hard to digest and inflammation producing, which is why I'll be asking you to omit them for now (and to eliminate gluten permanently). See pages 86 to 88 for more.

Choose Organic—You Are Worthy!

When to invest in organic and when to let it slide? I'd love for us all to eat organic all the time (in the old days it was easy; organic was simply known as *food*). Nonorganic food, a.k.a. conventional food, is grown with pesticides designed to kill, can include hormones that can change ours, and can be genetically modified (altered from its natural state to get it to grow when otherwise it might not). The seeds are tampered with to make a bigger, shinier product—yet altered in ways we might not yet be aware of. That's a game with nature I'd prefer not to join.

When you look at "conventional" food that way, is it something you really want to eat? It's true that organic can be costlier, so it pays to figure out your options. Here is my organic priority list, meaning whenever it's available and possible, I choose organic:

- Dairy
- Meat
- Eggs
- Produce

DAIRY. Cows producing nonorganic dairy are often pumped up with growth hormones so they can produce more, cheaper milk. Our growing kids' and our aging body's hormones are constantly changing, sometimes in unpredictable ways. Do you want all those *extra* hormones? I'm asking you to lay off dairy for now, but if you do try reintroducing it (see page 136), make sure it's organic.

MEAT AND EGGS. Meat also can contain added hormones, and the animals are often treated with antibiotics. Those antibiotics are *preventive*, because the animals are designed to eat certain foods, but instead we're feeding them processed junk they can't digest and would otherwise make them sick (yes, sadly, animals eat processed junk, too). Conventionally raised chickens, both for meat and eggs, are also fed antibiotics because the horribly crowded cages they're kept in are a hotbed of disease.

PRODUCE. Fruits and vegetables can vary widely in how much they are sprayed. I rely on the Environmental Working Group (EWG; www.ewg.org) to update me with the latest "Dirty Dozen" list of the most highly sprayed produce. Make organic your priority there. To keep your expenses in check, focus on those twelve and go conventional with EWG's "Clean Fifteen." Another aging in reverse benefit: Organic produce is higher in disease-fighting antioxidants. These compounds protect the plant, and without all the pesticides, organic fruits and vegetables need to work harder so they make more antioxidants.

Here are some other ways to go organic on a budget:

- **Buy frozen organic fruits and vegetables.** They are generally less expensive and are frozen at the height of freshness, so you won't be compromising taste or nutrition.

- **Buy in bulk and freeze it.** As soon as you get home from the store or farmers' market, portion your food into freezer bags or containers and immediately put them in the freezer. Look for sales to increase your savings. Buy those berries and greens and freeze them for later.

- **Look for coupons online.** Be a smart Internet shopper. You'll be amazed by the savings out there.

- **Join a local food co-op.** Not only will you save money, but because co-ops often offer educational programs, talks, and cooking classes, becoming a member will help you with one of your mind-set goals, Add the Good (see page 30). It's a healthy way to meet people on a similar path.

- **Shop smart at the farmers' market.** Shopping local guarantees freshness and amazing choices, but the food is often costlier than in the grocery store. Do a full round before committing to purchases so you're sure to come home with the best value and quality. Ask vendors whether their produce is organically grown and their meats are grass-fed. At the height of growing season, farmers often have excess and offer special deals. Vendors like to sell out, so if you go near closing time, you'll likely find lowered prices.

- **Grow your own.** Start small with a windowsill herb garden, and if you have the space, clear out a plot and get planting. A good garden center will share with you the tools and know-how to get started. If you don't have access to your own outdoor space, look for a shared community garden—another great way of meeting positive people and adding the good!

- **Use all parts of your food.** Save your parsley, cilantro, and other herb stems for juicing or to chop finely and add to stir-fries (read more about these Neglected Veggies on page 110). Or add them to your bone broth as it cooks, along with vegetable scraps you've saved from prepping. Add lemon, lime, or orange rinds to water to flavor it. Use the bones from yesterday's roast chicken as the base of tomorrow's bone broth.

FOCUS ON ABUNDANCE

This mind-set shift is can fuel your transformation journey. Having an attitude of gratitude will multiply your abundance. When you apply the concept to nutrition, it will keep you from obsessing about what you are missing and instead focused on what you are receiving.

Write down five new unprocessed foods you'd like to try, then start to incorporate them into your day. Curious about curcumin? Add a pinch of turmeric to your scrambled eggs. How about seaweed? Start cautiously by adding a strip of kombu (see page 108) to your bone broth to give it a flavor and nutrition boost. Or maybe it's an exotic fruit, such as goji berries. Anything unprocessed is fair game!

1. _____   3. _____   5. _____

2. _____   4. _____

There is another bonus to organic food: it tastes better. If you don't believe me, go ahead and do a side-by-side taste test! I did one with strawberries and raspberries with my husband and, hands down, he chose organic.

Make organic important to you, and you'll find a way. What can you let go of to make room for more organic? What you eat is the most determining factor in disease prevention, so why not make it a priority?

Consider the rule of addition versus subtraction. Earlier I talked about adding the good by surrounding yourself with positive people, reading inspiring books, and listening to educational podcasts and other talks (see pages 30 to 31). Now think about how much good you can add to your plate: *How many fresh vegetables and fruits can you add to your day? And how many of those can be organic?* Challenge yourself to eat the colors of the rainbow. *How much water can you drink throughout the day?* Check that off and you'll be less hungry and less bloated.

Instead of obsessing over what you *can't* eat, think of how much you can add. Picture plates brimming with veggies, probiotic-rich ferments, and anti-inflammatory superfoods set against a perfect balance of protein, carbs, and fats as your base. In the next chapter, we'll see what that looks like.

Take a Pause from Your Plate

Contrary to popular dietary trends, I'm not a fan of extremes in which you're eating just a few hours a day. The term *intermittent fasting* typically means all your food for the day is eaten in a small window, usually anywhere between four to six hours. This gives your body a rest from creating insulin so you can go into fat-burning mode. The problem: when you stop doing it, which you inevitably will, you're going to gain weight. If you could sustain this way of eating for a lifetime, that would be fine, but it just isn't feasible for most people. However, *small* cycles of fasting are hugely beneficial for our insulin levels. I recommend *modified fasting*, or taking a twelve-hour break from eating every day. That break is long enough for you to stop secreting insulin and put you into fat-burning mode every day, and is something completely doable for most of us. As a bonus, confining your eating to certain times almost automatically means you'll be eating less (no more midnight refrigerator raids!). I continue to

NUTRITION IS THE FUEL FOR EVERYTHING

Why does nutrition matter? Because it's where the majority of your results are. If you want to get serious about fat loss and long-term health, solely focusing on working out won't cut it. You've got to put most of your efforts into what you eat. Going unprocessed means not just eating from certain food categories but getting the right nutrients from the right foods. Without the right nutrition, no matter how much time you spend in the gym, you won't get the results you want.

How you fuel your body plays a huge role beyond fat loss. In fact, it is the most determining factor in our overall health, including prevention or reversal of type 2 diabetes and other diseases. Nutrition is key to our daily energy levels. It is so important that if you were to never work out again but still have good nutrition, you'd still see a transformation. Of course, that doesn't mean you should skip your workouts! You can always find examples of amazing athletes who eat whatever they want, including candy and junk. Their body is more forgiving, at least in the short term. But sound eating will carry you for your entire life. Note: A lot of us think we're athletes, but few of us actually are. There's a difference between being an Olympic swimmer and going to the gym for a few hours a week!

be a big advocate of breakfast, so my advice is to stop eating earlier so you can have your morning meal soon after waking up.

Keep Adding the Good

Eating unprocessed means eating in balance so you're not giving up entire food groups. You know what happens when you make dietary changes focused on deprivation. You start wanting those foods you gave up even more, you start craving them, and you feel like a failure when you give in, which you inevitably will. Instead, keep adding the good!

Making an unprocessed diet your base is the most effective way of maintaining your health, fighting disease, and losing fat and keeping it off. No matter what dietary plan you're following, you can benefit from adding more and more unprocessed foods to your diet at every point in your life.

EAT BEFORE YOU'RE HUNGRY

If you're already hungry by the time you sit down to eat, you're much more likely to overeat. When you learn to pay attention to your hunger naturally, you can eliminate hunger pangs and that feeling of being "starved" before your meals. Here are a few tips for keeping hunger at bay:

- Make sure your meals are balanced with the right amount of protein, carbs, and fat (see pages 69 to 74).

- Make sure you are eating enough.

- Don't consume artificial sweeteners (read more on pages 84 to 85).

- Cut back on starchy carbs and eliminate any lingering sugar.

- Enjoy a healthy snack before eating out to take the edge off.

- Drink a glass of water before your meals.

- If you know you're going to be famished by a certain time, eat sooner.

Step 3

Balance Your Plate with Protein, Fats, and Carbs

Despite conflicting information from an overwhelming number of diet gurus, making healthy food choices is simple. Plan your plate with the correct balance of macronutrients—protein, fats, and carbs—three meals a day (with unlimited veggies; see page 155) and you'll feel satisfied and empowered to make healthy choices going forward. Protein, fat, and carbs are the building blocks for your perfect meal and the perfect vehicle for fat loss and staying fit and healthy throughout your life. To balance your plate, you won't be counting calories. Rather, you'll be using your hand as a guide. It's really that simple! You'll soon be able to make everyday choices so you can build meals of your own design, even off a restaurant menu.

Protein

Protein is important for us at all times of our life, and it's particularly important for women, who tend not to get enough. When our hormones start to change, eating protein becomes even more essential, because this is the time when our body starts losing lean mass (see more on page 129). Protein builds lean muscle, which keeps our metabolism functioning at its best, and this is essential for weight loss and management. Protein also

WHAT ABOUT PROTEIN BARS?

Convenient? Yes. Healthy? Most brands are not. Protein bars are often higher in sugar than candy bars and full of junk. To stay true to its name, a protein bar should have three to four times the amount of protein as carbs, but this is often not the case. Another thing to consider is that the protein in these bars is typically coming from processed soy sources, such as soy protein isolate, and we want to avoid soy right now (more on page 133). Real food is always the ideal, but if your options are truly limited, look for a protein bar with ingredients you can define—simple, natural ingredients, such as eggs, nuts, seeds, and fruits. Or, even better, make your own using the recipe on page 237. Another option is 100 percent protein jerky. Look for jerky in a natural food store (not the gas station) made from grass-fed animals and that contains no added sugar.

supports our bones, hair, nails, and skin. Although dairy contains protein, I want you to avoid it for now (see pages 86 to 87) and focus on other animal protein, organic whenever possible.

Protein portion size:
the size of your fist, or 4 to 6 ounces, with each meal

See page 153 for a full list of proteins to choose from.

Fat

By now most of us have heard that fat is not the enemy. We need fat to live, and low-fat diets are doomed to fail. Fat helps us feel full and stay full and gives us long-lasting energy, as opposed to the quick bursts that sugar provides and that leave us feeling hungrier soon after. Healthy fats from such foods as avocado, olive oil, and nuts are brain food, and can help with memory and

VEGETABLE OILS—OR, DON'T BE FOOLED BY THE NAME

In the next chapter, I'll explain why it's so important to up your veggie intake. But when it comes to oils, it's best to avoid vegetable oils, and the same goes for soy, corn, and canola oils. Unlike heart-healthy extra-virgin olive oil and unrefined coconut oil, these oils are refined, which means they are stripped of their nutrients, color, flavor, and even aroma. That's why they all have the same bland taste, can keep on the shelf forever, and are very cheap. Contrast that to olive oil—each type has its own unique flavor and aroma—and unrefined coconut oil, which tastes like coconut. These are real, unprocessed oils that will feed your body and brain the fuel it needs to stay on top. You may also experiment with avocado oil (make sure the word *unrefined* is on the label here, too, as many brands are not) and nut and seed oils, such as macadamia oil and pumpkin seed oil. What about the omega-3 fatty acids canola oil is supposed to contain? Those have been denatured by the refining process, so not only are the benefits gone, but ingesting this refined oil can lead to the formation of carcinogenic free radicals, making a processed oil–rich diet a huge health concern. Remember: there's no place for trans fats *or* refined vegetable oils in an unprocessed foods diet.

cognition, reduce brain inflammation, and lower the risk of brain diseases, such as Alzheimer's. Fat also helps us absorb certain vitamins and joins forces with protein in its hair-, nail-, and skin-nourishing abilities. Fats to enjoy include oils, avocado, nuts, and seeds (make sure nuts and seeds are raw and unsalted). Note that nuts and seeds contain protein, but they're mostly fat, so that's why I've included them in this category. All oils must be unprocessed (look for the words *unrefined* or *extra-virgin* on the label; see sidebar). We'll be avoiding butter for now but enjoying ghee, a form of clarified butter with the milk solids removed. You can find ghee at natural food stores, or make your own using the recipe on page 168. Coconut milk from a can counts as a fat, but other nut milks do not because their fat content is minimal.

> **Fat portion size: the size of your thumb,
> or 1 to 2 tablespoons, with each meal**

See page 154 for a full list of healthy fats to choose from.

Carbohydrates

For the purpose of this plan, there are only two types of carbs that I want you to pay attention to and that count as part of your total daily allowance. Those are carbs from the starchy carb family (such as sweet potatoes and corn) and most fruit (fresh, frozen, freeze-dried, and dried). The exceptions are fresh strawberries, blueberries, raspberries, and blackberries. You do not have to count these berries because they are so low in carbs and sugar that they can be eaten in unlimited quantities the way vegetables can be eaten!

It's very much worth it to do a simple mathematical equation and a little number crunching to look and feel your best for a long, long time. For a total of five carb counts per day, you may enjoy up to two starchy carbs servings and anywhere from three to five fruit carbs, depending on your starchy carb consumption for the day.

If you consume two starchy carb counts in any one day, you may also have three fruit servings. If you have fewer than two starchy carbs, you may have more fruit carbs to make up the difference. Remember, it is one carb serving per meal and up to two snacks. This means if you include a starchy carb in a meal or snack, do not also include a fruit carb in that meal.

Here's a few examples of what your daily carb count should look like for you:

> **2 starchy carbs + 3 fruit carbs = 5 carbs total**
> **1 starchy carbs + 4 fruit carbs = 5 carbs total**
> **0 starchy carbs + 5 fruit carbs = 5 carbs total**

Vegetables are also carbs, but they are nonstarchy and considered unlimited on this plan as long as they are raw or steamed. That means you don't have to measure them! In fact, I'd like veggies to make up the majority of your plate. Veggies are nutrient dense, fiber rich, and low in calories (read more about why you should be eating more of them in the next chapter). They do not need to be combined with protein and fat. Note that corn (the vegetable, not the grain) and potatoes both count as starchy carbs, not vegetables. And don't worry about carrots and beets—yes, they are sweeter than other vegetables, but they're still vegetables with lots of nutrients. No one ever got fat by eating too many carrots or beets! As I mentioned earlier, because they are so low in sugar (and high in nutrients), blackberries, raspberries, blueberries, and strawberries are also considered unlimited.

Starchy carb portion size:
Starchy carbs are the size of your fist, or ½ cup.

See page 154 for a full list of starchy carbs to choose from.

STOP THE VICIOUS STARCHY CARB CYCLE

Always combine proteins, fats, and carbs to build your daily meals, but proteins or fats can be eaten on their own as snacks. Whenever you eat a carb, though, pairing it with a fat or a protein is a must. If you eat starchy carbs, such as potatoes, on their own, you'll likely get a blood sugar spike. When your blood sugar spikes, your body secretes insulin, which is followed by a dip that leaves you with lower blood sugar. You need that fat and protein to balance you out, otherwise cravings and overeating inevitably ensue. Let's stop that vicious carb cycle!

What if you're eating the proper balance and you're still hungry? Increase your protein and put V3 (see the next chapter) into high gear! I've planned ten days of meals following this formula (see pages 158 to 162) to get you started. After the ten-day mark, you'll see how easy it is to create your daily meals going forward.

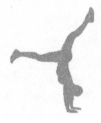

Step 4

Pack Your Plate with V3:
Value, Volume, Vegetables!

People are always looking for a magic pill. The one that will finally give them more energy. The one that will make them look and feel younger. The one that will help them realize their fat-loss goals. The one that will give them the most bang for their buck. The good news is there is one! Vegetables and more of them are just what *everybody* needs for protection against the growing list of toxic substances found in our environment and the standard American (a.k.a. processed) diet. Vegetables are filled with fiber and are low in calories, they keep you regular, give you energy, improve your complexion, boost your

HOW TO GET IN YOUR GREENS

To ensure you're getting in lots of greens every day, my ten-day meal plan includes a daily Super Salad (page 227) based on leafy greens and enriched with superfoods (see pages 104 to 118) to further nourish you. Try it for ten days, then see whether you can commit to a Super Salad every day going forward.

mood, and may even reduce your risk of cancer, diabetes, and heart disease. Vegetables are supremely hydrating. Foods that are fortified with vitamins and minerals are trying to make up for lack of the abundance found in vegetables. Because vegetables are the building blocks for preventing disease, there's no substitute for the real thing.

We've come a long way in our understanding of the importance of veggies. Before I was diagnosed with celiac disease, I went to a gastroenterologist who actually suggested I eat more bread and pasta and to give up vegetables. He thought veggies were contributing to the painful bloating that was in reality caused by the erosion of the villi in my stomach from eating gluten. Now, fewer doctors would suggest such a course. Pale iceberg lettuce wedges have been replaced by cancer-fighting kale, potato no longer counts as a veggie, and current popular eating plans, from vegan to paleo, recommend that our plates be composed of at least half veggies. So, it's time to put into practice V3 and add veggie volume to every plate!

From asparagus to zucchini, enjoy a rainbow of veggies. Brightly colored vegetables are filled with anti-inflammatory phytonutrients, each with their unique phytonutrient profile. They are all superfoods (read more about them on pages 106 to 107). Cruciferous vegetables, including cauliflower, broccoli, Brussels sprouts, and cabbage, have been shown to have powerful anti-cancer qualities. Those benefits are multiplied when crucifers are eaten raw, which is good reason to add naturally fermented sauerkraut (see pages 96 to 97) and raw cauliflower rice (see the box on page 177) to your diet.

DEVELOP A VEGGIE-CENTRIC MIND-SET

Put into action two concepts you learned in Change Your State—Create New Habits (page 40) and Add the Good (page 30)—by committing to adding more veggies to your life. See how good you feel when veggies are the main event rather than an afterthought!

Sprouts are a concentrated veggie delivery system, as they are bursting with vitamins, minerals, antioxidants, and live enzymes. They have up to thirty times the nutrients of their mature vegetable counterparts and are extremely low in calories. It's easy to sprout in your own kitchen and it costs pennies per cup to make. Look for sprouting kits in natural food stores or online.

Use the list on page 155 to compose your veggie shopping list and turn to page 145 for prep tips to shortcut your way to three meals a day of V3.

A PLANT-BASED DIET

The term *plant-based* means different things to different people, but mostly it's equated with eating a vegan diet. To me, plant-based is simply that the bulk of your food comes from a plant, meaning a vegetable or fruit. Even though I am not vegan or vegetarian, I still consider my diet plant-based because I practice the principles of V3.

In any plan, we need a balance of nutrients, and vegetarians and vegans in particular want to pay particular attention to protein. Adding grains and beans to your diet will increase your protein, but it will also make your diet carb heavy, and a primarily carb-based diet could lead to weight gain and work against that lean physique you're after. If you're a vegetarian, you'd have to eat a fair amount of eggs and supplement with protein powder to balance your plate in the proportions that work for my plan and it's even more difficult to sustain my plan as a vegan. For those reasons, my meal plan does not offer vegetarian or vegan options.

HOW TO GET MORE VEGGIES INTO YOUR LIFE

- Ask to sub veggies for pasta, grains, or potato when you're eating out.

- Cook veggies into bone broth (page 163).

- Blend veggies into soups (pages 222 to 226) and smoothies (pages 190 to 195).

- Munch on carrot and celery sticks.

- Learn to ferment veggies (page 174 and 231) or buy live pickles or sauerkraut from the store.

- Make 100 percent vegetable juice.

- Snack on veggie hummus (page 233).

- Puree veggies; a pound of cooked spinach blends down to about a cup, enabling you to really pack in the V3.

- Start a kale chip habit.

- Eat a Super Salad (page 227) every day.

- Pack veggies into single-serving packets so they're always at arm's reach.

- Stock up on packets of freeze-dried veggie snacks for when you're traveling.

Step 5

Keep Your Plate Clear of Added Sugar (and Its Artificial Imitators) and Slow Down on Starchy Carbs

Sugar is possibly the most inflammatory—and addictive—substance most people eat every single day. It's no wonder the average American eats about 130 pounds of sugar a year. We start "using" as kids and fast-track to a sweet tooth that can't be satisfied and that ultimately leaves our body bloated and in danger of getting type 2 diabetes, a disease that is hitting people at a younger age than ever.

Eliminating sugar, even natural forms of the sweet stuff, could be the biggest step you take to combat the effects of inflammation, one of the biggest contributors to disease as we age. Even if it's honey, brown sugar, maple syrup, coconut sugar, or agave nectar, in the end it's still added sugar, and it's not serving any purpose beyond feeding our desire to have more. While these options might be healthier, they still can trigger cravings.

It's more important than ever to avoid sugar while experiencing hormonal changes (see more on the subject on page 132). I'd like you to eliminate *all* sweeteners as you work through the plan, and once you are in maintenance mode, you can start adding back natural sweeteners in small portions. And since starchy carbs break down into sugar, they are one step away from adding to the journey of destruction that sugar makes through your body.

A Sugar and Starchy Carb Nightmare

What happens when we eat too many sugary sweets or starchy carbs, such as bread, cookies, crackers, and packaged snack foods? Fasten your seatbelt, because I'm going to share a little science with you here.

When we eat carbs, they are broken down and absorbed into our bloodstream as the sugar glucose, which in turn elevates our blood sugar levels. This signals the release of insulin, a hormone produced by the pancreas. Insulin's main job is to regulate blood sugar levels by getting sugar out of the blood and into cells to use for energy, or to the liver or muscles to be turned into glycogen and stored for later.

When we eat too many carbs, especially processed carbs made from white flour and sugar, a big spike in insulin secretion follows. Since insulin's job is to lower blood sugar, it does just that. But because of that insulin spike, your blood sugar gets lowered too much, and this is when you crash. You know, that feeling you get after a big bowl of pasta, oatmeal sweetened with sugar, or a second slice of cake. The nonscientific term for this state is *food coma*. These spikes and crashes wreak havoc with insulin, not only leaving you with that groggy, cranky feeling, but increasing your risk for diabetes and other chronic diseases.

And what about when your body already has enough energy? Energy can be stored for later, but if the glycogen stores in your muscles and liver are full, then the excess blood sugar is stored as body fat. If your body is secreting insulin, it is in a "storing" process, and no body fat will be burned.

To cut to the chase: When your body is producing insulin, you're not in fat-burning mode. For this reason, you want to eliminate added sugar and processed carbs so you can minimize insulin spikes and keep them on an even keel.

And it's not just weight gain and insulin responses that you need to be concerned about. When you're in perimenopause or menopause, sugary and starchy carbs go a step further, increasing your risk for depression. Eating foods that are high on the glycemic index (that is, foods that send your blood sugar soaring and crashing, such as pasta and white bread) have been shown to be a risk factor for depression in postmenopausal women.

This could be because these foods increase inflammation, insulin resistance, and risk of heart disease, all of which can lead to depression, or it could be because the constant up and down of blood sugar messes with your brain and mood.

We're not done yet. Starchy and sugary carbs can be a nightmare for bones, too. High-sugar diets have been shown to lower bone mineral density and bone strength, possibly because an abundance of insulin makes it harder for the body to hang on to calcium. The worst part: Research shows this is an even bigger problem for women. Since bone density is already a concern during hormonal shifts, now is the time to give up the sugar and processed carbs for good.

Going very low carb might seem like the logical fix and can even be a temporary solution. You'll dig into your glycogen stores for energy and lose weight at first. The problem is, your body and brain need carbohydrates to function. Eventually you will need carbs again. It's all about choosing the right carbs. I recommend limiting starchy carbs (see page 154) but not eliminating carbs altogether. We'll talk about the right carbohydrates choices later on.

IF YOU DO INDULGE

If you eat a high-sugar or -carbohydrate meal, make sure you eat plenty of fiber and balance it out with protein and fat. That way the sugar will hit your bloodstream more slowly, you won't get as much of an insulin spike or the inevitable sugar low that follows, and you're more likely to be satisfied by a single indulgence without reaching for seconds or thirds. For example, instead of a giant fruit smoothie for breakfast, make it a smaller smoothie with scrambled eggs and avocado on the side.

Don't Aim High with Fructose
(but Keep Eating Fruit!)

Sugar, no matter what form it is in, is by far one of the most dangerous substances that you can eat. But when it's in the form of high-fructose corn syrup (HFCS), it is even worse. Fructose, as its name implies, is the sugar found in fruit. So, is fruit making us fat? No! Fruit is healthy for us in its original form because it has a built-in mechanism called fiber that prevents its sugars from overloading the liver and supports our health with vital minerals, vitamins, and antioxidants, which table sugar could never dream of doing.

The culprit is HFCS. If you've ever read a label, you're probably familiar with HFCS. It's in most processed foods from cereal, muffins, and crackers, to ketchup and soda. It's everywhere because it's cheaper than sugar. That it's based on genetically modified corn is enough to make you want to steer clear of the substance. But that it overloads our liver is equally alarming. Remember, all cells in our body can metabolize glucose. But the only organ that can metabolize fructose is the liver. So, when we eat a diet high in HFCS, the liver gets overloaded. The fructose is coming in so fast the liver doesn't know what to with it and starts turning the fructose into fat. Not only does this fat end up in our thighs and belly, the backs of our arms, and hips, but this fat also builds up in our liver. When we force our liver to synthesize fats, it causes fat around our organs and can bring on high blood pressure, heart disease, leaky gut, and insulin resistance, which can lead to obesity and type 2 diabetes. In addition, HFCS slows down the secretion of the hormone leptin in the body. Why is this important? Because leptin is in charge of sending signals to our body to indicate that we are full. That's why a diet high in HFCS—today's processed diet—leads to overeating. The equation is simple: cheap food causes overconsumption and addiction, which can lead to weight gain, diabetes, heart disease, and other diseases. The only winners are the companies that make these products.

HOW TO BEAT CRAVINGS

Cravings are a huge stumbling block to fat loss, and willpower alone is never enough to sustain lasting change. When you make a decision to cut out certain foods (in particular, foods containing sugar), your body initially wants those foods back. Most people try to willpower their way out of those cravings. But no matter how strong-willed you are, if you are fighting cravings every single day at every single meal, it is easy to get discouraged and give up. That's why sticking to a new way of eating can be challenging. And that's why you have to balance every plate you plan. And never forget your driving core motivator (see page 25), the reason why you are doing all this in the first place.

With all my years of eating unprocessed under my belt, I still get triggered when I make slight mistakes. For example, I recently made a berry pie. I used gluten-free flour, agave nectar as a sweetener, and organic berries. It didn't matter. I ate one slice of the pie, put it away, then got up to get another slice. I got up again and again until I literally polished off the entire pie. After a temporary high, I crashed. Even this licensed master sports nutritionist was no match for pie! I would have been better off skipping the pie altogether and instead eating a bowl of fresh berries (perhaps topped with a spoonful of Coconut Whipped Cream—see page 181 for the recipe), because one bite was all it took for those cravings to kick in.

The good news is that while carbohydrates and sugar stimulate the production of insulin, fats and proteins do not. That's why it's critical to combine carbs with fats and protein and to build your meal in the perfect proportion of the three (see page 69). Think of fat and protein as your dynamic duo. They give you the superpower of will-power because you'll feel full and will no longer need to turn to sugar for another short-lived energy boost.

CARB ALERT!
BEWARE THE STEADY RELEASE OF INSULIN

When you nibble on carbohydrate-rich snack foods, and especially when they contain no added fat, your body steadily releases insulin. This causes your blood sugar to lower, which in turn tells you to keep eating to get it back up. Now you know why you just couldn't put those fat-free crackers, chips, and cookies down!

Steer Clear of Artificial Sweeteners

Maybe you've kicked the sugar habit and swapped in artificial sweeteners to get your fix. Maybe it's just a daily diet soda or sugar-free gum. You think you're doing something good by avoiding the calories, but then you're craving more and not feeling great. That's because your body is getting tricked. When your body senses the sweetness, it asks, "Where are the calories?" That's when you start eating even *more* calories elsewhere to make up for this deprivation. Food manufacturers would like you to believe that sugar-free snacks are the have-your-cake-and-eat-it-too answer to dieting. But nothing could be further from the truth.

Most artificial sweeteners, from the original, saccharine, to aspartame, sucralose (Splenda), sorbitol, mannitol, and xylitol, are anywhere from two hundred to six hundred times sweeter than sugar. Imagine how this can mess with your taste buds! Then when you eat a natural sweet, such as fruit, it no longer tastes sweet. To top it off, artificial sweeteners can have other side effects, from bloating to digestive issues, nausea, migraines, and even brain tumors. And they can kick hormonal issues into high gear, the last thing any woman wants! Eating these sweeteners can throw your appetite-regulating hormones out of whack, which in turn throws off your hunger and fullness cues and leads to overeating. They can also mess with insulin release, alter the microbiome in your gut, and ultimately impair your entire metabolism and cause you to gain weight.

So, although these low-calorie sweets may be tempting, they are not helping you with your health goals. My recommendation is to stay clear of *all* artificial sweeteners. Give your taste buds time to get back in the game, so a sweet potato tastes sweet again and fruit is a satisfying treat. If you can't do without sweetener in your daily beverages, try stevia, derived from a South American plant. Stevia is completely natural and up to three hundred times sweeter than sugar, but has negligible effects on blood sugar. Look for stevia leaf extract in the least processed powder or liquid form.

THE DIET SODA CONNECTION

A decade ago, my mother was having severe migraines. She went to a number of specialists, took migraine medications, and nothing was working. Until she stopped drinking diet soda. As soon as she eliminated that source of artificial sweetener, her migraines went away. Some researchers have found aspartame and sucralose to be triggers for migraines, all the more reason to eliminate *all* diet sodas and artificial sweeteners from your diet.

Step 6

Clear Your Plate of Inflammation Triggers

After recovery from surgery for the mother of all ruptured discs, part of my comeback involved clearing my plate of lingering inflammation triggers. I'd already gone gluten free years back, after my celiac diagnosis, but with the stakes even higher, I went deeper into reducing inflammation and clearing my digestion by eliminating grains, beans, and legumes from my diet. And because dairy is mucus producing and can contribute to inflammation, eliminating dairy as well became the missing link for me.

Ditch the Dairy

The lactose (milk sugar) and protein (casein) can be difficult to digest for many people. If you are someone who is allergic to casein, you have no choice but to avoid all dairy products. Many of us lose our ability to digest lactose (lactose intolerance) at some point in our lives, and eating dairy products can cause a mild to major reaction, from gas to bloating, stomach pains, and diarrhea. In some cases, fermented dairy products, such as yogurt and kefir, can be tolerated, as the fermentation removes most of the lactose. And as most of the lactose is removed from butter to make ghee, ghee can be enjoyed by many people who cannot otherwise eat dairy (see my recipe on page 168).

When our digestive system is in top shape, we can enjoy a wide range of foods including dairy. Unfortunately, thanks to processed foods, dairy from cows fed genetically modified food, and a stressful lifestyle, in addition to the inevitable inflammation, our digestion typically runs into problems, most typically leaky gut, at some point in our lives and especially as we age (see more on leaky gut on page 89). For many of us, dairy is a top trigger, and it often goes hand in hand with gluten.

If you just can't say no to pizza, a cheese sandwich, or cake, that's because they are, quite literally, comfort foods: scientists have found traces of morphinelike substances that have opioid-like effects, in both gluten and dairy. Many people who have celiac disease also are lactose intolerant. Avoiding gluten *and* dairy can quickly reduce inflammation. It did the trick for me, and I'd like you to try it while you're following this plan. Take care when reading package labels for hidden dairy (it sneaks into foods you wouldn't expect!), and for your tea, coffee, and smoothies, nut milks make a delicious dairy-free stand-in. Learn how to make your own nut milk on page 167.

It is possible for some of us to enjoy dairy again once we've repaired our gut. The only way to know is to reintroduce it. If and when you're ready, start with fermented dairy, such as yogurt or kefir, and go for raw milk dairy if possible. Make sure any dairy you eat is organic. Read more about reintroducing foods on page 136.

Get Rid of Grains, Be Done with Beans, and Lose the Legumes

While grains contain fiber, vitamins, and minerals, they can also be a challenge to your digestion, exacerbate leaky gut, and cause on-the-spot fatigue and bloat. Taking a break from grains while removing gluten completely from your diet is just what your body needs to quell the flames of inflammation and lose the lingering fat. For your starchy carbs, beta-carotene-rich sweet potatoes, moderate amounts of white potatoes, fresh corn, and delicious fruits will satisfy without triggering the cravings that lead you to reach for seconds and thirds.

It's common knowledge and the butt of many jokes that beans can be hard to digest. They act similarly to grains in how they are digested and typically do not offer the same nutritional profile as animal sources. Most soy is genetically modified and overly processed and contains phytoestrogens, which mimic natural estrogen. As our hormones start to change, it's generally not a good idea to eat foods that can potentially raise our estrogen levels (see the box on page 95).

Grains, beans, and legumes contain antinutrients, such as phytic acid, in their outer layer or bran; and untreated, it can bind to the minerals calcium, magnesium, copper, iron, and zinc and block their absorption from your body. They also contain enzyme inhibitors, which can impede digestion. This can put a strain on the digestive system, and some health experts believe this is part of the cause of sensitivities and intolerances toward them. Simply soaking for a few hours and then discarding the soaking water neutralizes these antinutrients, and this is what I recommend you do if you would like to try adding them back to your diet (see page 136). Because white rice does not contain a layer of bran, it is more digestible for some people.

CUT OUT THE GLUTEN

I talked extensively about gluten and my journey to discovering I had celiac disease in my first book, *Natalie Jill's 7-Day Jump Start*. Gluten is the protein found in wheat, rye, and barley, and celiac disease is an autoimmune disorder in which the body does not recognize gluten and responds with symptoms ranging from stomach pains to skin rashes and gets progressively worse. The only way to get rid of the symptoms is to give up gluten entirely. Even if you haven't been diagnosed with celiac disease, I still recommend eliminating gluten from your diet, especially as you age and enter menopause. Here's why:

Celiac disease affects a small percentage of the people, but some researchers suggest gluten sensitivity may be more common than first realized. And, you guessed it, intolerances and sensitivities are more common in women. Our body is vulnerable to the toxic effects of gluten, likely because modern wheat is much higher in gluten and our gastrointestinal and immune systems have not adapted to handle this.

Gluten is a trigger for inflammation and has been shown to cause an immune response in many people. Our gut recognizes the protein as an invader, so we produce antibodies to attack it (for people with celiac disease, the situation is even worse, as our immune system also attacks the enzyme we make that breaks gluten down).

One of the biggest problems that people with gluten sensitivity run into is a condition called leaky gut syndrome. Leaky gut occurs as a result of the development of gaps between the cells that make up the membrane lining your intestinal wall, which basically means the gut becomes permeable and substances, even toxic substances, can slip through the cracks and into the blood. In sensitive people, gluten is a major cause of this condition, causing bloat and discomfort, promoting inflammation, and speeding up the aging process.

Cutting out gluten has also been shown to improve bone mineral density, a factor we know is important during times of hormonal change. Even though some people can eat gluten without having an immune response or other negative side effects, I still say your best bet is to cut it out completely.

Unprocessed foods—fruits, vegetables, nuts, seeds, and meat— are gluten-free by nature, so eating unprocessed means there's no room for gluten in your diet. If you're wondering whether you should go gluten-free, ask yourself whether you should be on an unprocessed foods diet, and if you ask me, the answer is an unequivocal yes! See how you feel after not eating gluten for a few days; chances are, even if you don't find you have an intolerance, you will have more energy and will feel better.

ARE YOU FEELING TIRED AND BLOATED?

Wondering what might be draining your energy? Ask yourself the following questions:

- **Are you relying on caffeine to pull you through?** This temporary stimulant can come back to haunt you at bedtime.
- **Do any processed foods or sugar remain in your diet?** These culprits tend to spike your insulin and then create a countereffect that makes you feel more sluggish.
- **Are you getting in your V3?** If you aren't nourished with produce, your energy levels will be low. Upping fruits and vegetables is an easy way to get more energy right now. If making veggies the majority of your plate is a challenge, try taking a greens supplement (see page 124).

What causes belly bloat? These are the major culprits:

- Monthly hormonal swings and perimenopause/menopause (see page 126)
- Artificial sweeteners (see page 84)
- Dairy (lactose; see page 86)
- Wheat (gluten), other grains, beans, and legumes (see page 87)
- Other food intolerances and sensitivities
- Being dehydrated

Write down what you eat in your food log (page 149) and also make notes of when you feel bloated. You'll be able to connect the dots more easily when you see in black and white what you ate just prior to feeling tired or bloated. Are you more tired or bloated at certain times of the day? Are you eating lactose? Gluten? Is it processed? The body tends to respond to dairy, gluten, and grains and beans in general by retaining water (which is also what it does when you are dehydrated—it hangs on to every bit of moisture!). How did you feel in comparison when you did not eat those foods? Do you notice any trends?

Transformation

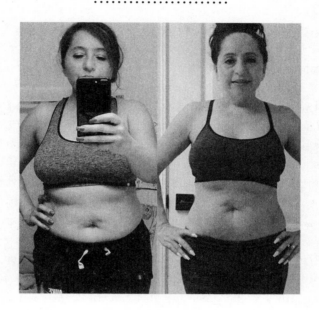

SUSANA

"My Shoulder Pain Disappeared After Giving Up Grains and Dairy"

I found Natalie Jill for the first time in 2014, when my husband and I did the 7-Day Jump Start to prepare for our honeymoon in Hawaii. We wanted to make some changes to our diet and get in shape, and we each lost about 8 pounds. Then, we started our own business and our priorities changed. All of our focus went to the business. I am in sales, and would have to carry five different phone books from office to office. It was taking its toll on my back. I gained some of the weight back and my back pain became so intense that eventually I had to go on medical leave.

I felt like a victim for an entire year. Then, I turned to Natalie again. The 7-Day Jump Start worked, so I thought I'd give her new program a try. I wanted to lose weight, but I got much more than I signed up for. The eating part was easy because the plan was clear, but what really worked for me was the mind-set piece. Natalie's questions got me to go deep. She encouraged me to ask myself, "Why am I a victim?" I had been making excuses for three years, and Natalie didn't put up with any of it. So it became impossible to keep coming up with excuses. When my mental state changed, my victim mode lifted. I was one of those people who thought the vision board was lame, and now I'm on my third after everything on the first and second vision boards became realities. My driving core motivator was my two-year-old grandson. I wanted to be able to pick him up and get stronger for him.

When I started the Aging in Reverse program, I noticed a huge increase in energy and focus and the pain remaining in my shoulder went away. I hadn't slept on my right side in two years because of tendinitis, and now that's no longer an issue. I attribute it to giving up grains and dairy. Making that dietary shift worked so much better than the ibuprofen my doctor told me to take. The menus were realistic, the recipes give lots of options, and the protein bites, fudge, and crackers have been a lifeline. They gave me a sense of having familiar foods. I lost an additional 5 pounds, in addition to the 11 pounds I lost in the previous program, and I am down to a size 4. I won't go back to grains and dairy because all I can think of is my shoulder pain returning. I'm living proof that eating this way can change your life. At forty-eight, I feel like I can keep getting better. I can say it a thousand times because the truth never changes!

I had been afraid to fail, so I would make small goals. But Natalie taught me that setting goals, reaching them, then setting new goals keeps you engaged. I love Natalie's simple yet powerful message that we are the only ones who limit ourselves. I didn't know that with my weight loss would come pain loss, more confidence, and a booming business!

Step 7

Perk Up Your Plate with Fermented Foods

When you hear the term *fermented foods*, what comes to mind? If you're only thinking of sauerkraut or alcoholic beverages, I'm going to ask you to expand your horizons and get acquainted with one of the healthiest and most delicious types of food you can eat.

Fermented foods have held a special place in traditional diets all over the world, from Korea to Iceland and Germany. And if you've ever eaten a dill pickle, that's a product of good old American fermentation. While the industrial (processed) food system got us away from fermentation, the practice is experiencing a comeback that's picking up more and more steam as more and more people are realizing its health benefits. The flavors fermentation brings to your plate are diverse—from salty to tangy, sour, and tart—and the health benefits are numerous.

What are fermented foods? In the most basic sense, fermentation happens by letting a food sit out; as it sits, bacteria and yeasts feed on the nutrients in food, which creates lactic acid, which in turn transforms the taste and sometimes the texture of the food. After this process is complete, not only is the original food preserved—think of turning cabbage into sauerkraut—but the end result is also chock-full of probiotics. When you consume fermented foods, you're filling your body with higher levels of nutrients than the original version, in an easier-to-digest format.

While the word *bacteria* might summon up less than favorable connotations for some of us, they are not only beneficial, but completely necessary for the health of your gut. Eating fermented foods means you're working to maintain or repair the delicate balance of your gut so you can absorb your nutrients better and more efficiently. Fermented foods are one of nature's most powerful medicines, and recent research shows a compelling connection between gut health and overall health and even fat loss. It goes beyond digestion to the whole body-mind system.

We may think we're alone in our body. But actually our body teams up with trillions and trillions of bacteria and microbes that make up the balance of our gut and digestive system. Without them, we wouldn't be able to digest or metabolize our food as we were meant to. So, these microbes are truly beneficial to our overall health. You may be wondering, *Don't these bacteria naturally exist in our food anyway? Why do I have to purposely seek outside fermented foods?* Unfortunately, the reason they are making a reappearance in our modern-day diets is that they have largely gotten the boot from the standard American diet. Processed foods, empty white carbs (such as pasta), and a typical diet of sugar-laden treats means most of us are not getting the probiotics and enzymes our ancestors naturally consumed far more of. Modern processed foods have stripped our gut of beneficial bacteria, and eating fermented foods is the easiest way of regaining what we've lost. We can turn to supplements, of course, which I do recommend as insurance (see pages 119 to 125), but the fact remains that getting our nutrients from food is always most effective.

By keeping your body infused with probiotics, common digestive ailments, such as irritable bowel syndrome, can start to heal and your immune system will start to strengthen. Probiotics are also an ally in your weight-loss goals. It only makes sense that keeping your gut in check will have a positive effect on your cravings. Studies are showing more and more that probiotic-rich diets can knock out cravings for carbs and junky foods before they begin. When your gut is healthy, you absorb more nutrients from the foods you're getting, your body starts to self-regulate, and you have fewer cravings. Speaking of cravings, when you're looking for a sugar fix, turn to a salty ferment,

CHANGING HORMONES AND THE GUT

Gut microbiota (the bacteria in your gut) are influenced by—you guessed it—hormones. Estrogen in particular may be able to alter the balance of gut microbiota, and there is evidence of a decline in the number and variety of healthful bacteria in the gut in menopausal women. Gut bacteria are closely linked to the development of certain diseases, so this could explain why autoimmune diseases, such as lupus and arthritis, are more prevalent in women than in men. The link between lower estrogen levels and altered gut microbiota is likely also responsible for weight gain and fat distribution during menopause. In addition to eating an unprocessed diet, focusing on eating probiotic-rich foods, such as ferments, and getting in prebiotic fiber via fruits and vegetables can help support a healthy gut at all times of life.

such as a pickle or sauerkraut. A bite or two is enough to steer your taste buds savory.

If these benefits aren't enough, fermented foods are inexpensive to buy and even more inexpensive to make and they don't require any specialized knowledge, ingredients, or equipment. The cabbage and sea salt used to make sauerkraut cost just a fraction of what a vitamin shop would charge for a supplement. By fermenting your own food—turning cucumbers into pickles, for example—you are greatly extending the shelf life of the food. And because fermentation acts as a natural preservative for your food, you'll save money because you won't be tossing out foods as frequently.

Since the probiotics found in fermented foods keep your digestive enzymes working top notch, introducing more and more of them into your diet will cause your need for store-bought supplements to decline. Because probiotics assist your digestive system in absorbing more nutrients from your food, you won't necessarily have to rely on a daily multiple because you'll be

ANTIBIOTICS AND YOUR INTERNAL BACTERIA BALANCE

If you've taken antibiotics lately, you have thrown off your body's balance of bacteria. Ever take a round and then wind up with a yeast infection? Antibiotics work by killing off bacteria in the body: the bad *and* the good. So, after you finish a round of antibiotics, it is more essential than ever to replenish your body by eating lots of yummy fermented, probiotic-rich foods and supplementing as necessary.

getting exactly what you need from your diet. And, ultimately, that is the goal of an unprocessed diet.

There's a fermented food for just about every palate and every meal, and you can easily make any of these right in your kitchen and easily find them in stores.

There are a number of delicious ferments that you can add to your diet right now. Here are a few:

YOGURT: A glance at a good-quality carton and you'll see billions of live cultures on the label. Yogurt is rich in probiotics and active cultures and is a huge boost to your gut and overall health. There are a lot of dairy-free options made in a similar way—including coconut and almond—which I'd like you to favor for now while you're avoiding dairy. Always read labels for extra sugar and additives and choose a plain version of yogurt. If you'd like to dress up your yogurt, do it yourself with fruit, nuts, and coconut.

SAUERKRAUT: Sauerkraut contains two ingredients: chopped cabbage and salt, but the benefits belie its simplicity. Cabbage is a crucifer, and all crucifers have powerful antioxidant and anticancer properties. Fermentation increases those properties. See my recipe on page 174 if you'd like to give DIY a try.

SHOPPING FOR FERMENTS

Look for sauerkraut, pickles, and other fermented vegetables in your supermarket's cold case with the words *live, raw,* or *contains living cultures* on the label. Pass on anything that's on the shelf, as it's likely pasteurized and contains no living cultures. And when you get your ferments home, don't heat them or their enzymes will no longer be live.

Add sauerkraut to salads, put a little on your plate to add a pop of flavor, or snack on it by the forkful. Sauerkraut is a free food, meaning you can eat as much of it as you like.

KIMCHI: This Korean ferment is also based on cabbage—here napa cabbage—with added spices and usually carrots, scallions, and daikon radish. Eating kimchi on a regular basis can help with weight loss, boost the glow of your skin, and can even maintain colon health. Some packaged kimchi contains sugar, so read labels carefully. Kimchi is a free food, meaning you can eat as much of it as you like.

PICKLES: Nothing satisfies like a dill pickle brimming with life-giving probiotics. But sadly, most pickles are cooked with vinegar and added sugar and are pasteurized to make them shelf stable. A real dill pickle is made the old-fashioned way, through fermentation. Learn how to make them on page 231. It's a fast, easy, and delicious entry into fermentation! Pickles are a free food, meaning you can eat as many of them as you like.

KOMBUCHA: If you're a fan of drinking your probiotics, kombucha is a popular and increasingly available choice that helps with digestion and detoxing the body. Kombucha is a sweetened tea that's packed with beneficial bacteria and yeasts; fermentation is activated via a starter called a SCOBY (short for "symbiotic culture of bacteria and yeast") by feeding sugar to the tea. Most of the sugar is eaten through fermentation, but make sure to read labels. A kombucha made with mango is likely to have a higher sugar content than one made with berries or a plain one.

CIDER VINEGAR: Raw cider vinegar is great for helping regulate blood pressure and diabetes, and even aids in fat loss, and you only need a small amount of it. It's a great daily addition to your diet. Add a little to soups, salads, drinks, and salad dressing, and remember not to heat it to keep its live properties live. A spoonful mixed with water can chase away a sugar craving.

CHEESE: As you're avoiding dairy for now, try my cultured Creamy Cashew Cheese (page 170). If you decide to try reintroducing dairy to your diet, favor raw and unpasteurized cheeses (and make sure they're organic), as only these contain probiotics. You can find raw versions of goat's milk, sheep's milk, and even some cow's milk cheeses.

Step 8

Hydrate Your Plate

Hydration is your secret weapon for weight loss. We *are* water, as our body and brain are made up primarily of H_2O. It's no wonder that so many people who are constantly feeling tired or hungry are actually chronically dehydrated. Just increasing your hydration can make a huge difference in your hunger levels. Everything works better when you're properly hydrated. Water cleanses everything out, restores your energy, and is great for your skin and digestive system. Favor filtered water or mineral water to ensure the purity of this all-important form of hydration.

DRINK BEFORE YOU EAT

Try drinking a whole glass of water before every meal. You'll feel fuller more quickly and you'll likely eat less, giving a boost to your weight-loss efforts. If you're hungry between meals, drink some water before snacking to keep your portions in check (try my Super Water, page 165).

And it's not just what you're drinking, but also what you're eating. Build your plate around V3: value, volume, veggies (page 75), so you're never thirsty, and supplement with soups, salads, and fruit and veggie snacks so you can to eat your way to hydration. And, of course, drink water throughout the day. The ideal amount is eight to ten glasses, but if you are hydrating your plate, it can be a little less. If you find drinking water to be a chore, add a squeeze of lemon or lime, a slice or two of cucumber, or change it up with unflavored sparkling water or Super Water (page 165). And don't forget that smoothies (pages 190 to 195), 100 percent veggie juices, and bone broth (see page 163 for my homemade version) count as liquid hydration.

The idea is to not overhydrate but to constantly enjoy hydrating foods so you avoid getting thirsty—which you may mistake for hunger. And if you're a caffeine drinker, know that these beverages are actually dehydrating. When you have coffee or tea, drink extra water to make up for the deficit. Diet soda typically contains caffeine, but after learning about how artificial sweeteners can sabotage your weight-loss efforts and mess with your hormones (page 85), you kicked that habit to the curb, right?

GIVING GRATITUDE
FOR YOUR FIRST CUP

You start to get dehydrated while you sleep, so try bringing a full glass of water to your bedside before you tuck in. When you wake up, engage your mind-set with a moment of gratitude. So many people do not have access to clean water. Recognize your good fortune, empty the glass, and go forth with your day.

The Salt and Sodium Connection

If you need additional incentive to hydrate, consider that proper hydration as part of an unprocessed diet means good-bye to bloat. Your body no longer needs to retain water because it's getting ample supplies from outside. If you've been watching your salt to avoid bloat, be careful, because salt is a nonnegotiable nutrient that everyone needs to survive.

I'll share a story with you. A few years ago, I went on an 18-mile hike in the Grand Canyon. I had lots of water, my unprocessed protein bars, and bags of nuts, so I thought I was thoroughly prepared. I was doing fine, and then 10 miles in, I suddenly felt as if I was becoming dehydrated. I wondered what was going on. I thought, *Am I not in good enough shape?* I was drinking so much water, but by the time I reached the top, I was walking at a snail's pace and I didn't know whether I would make it. I got dizzy, threw up, and felt as though I had the flu. And then it dawned on me that my protein bars and nuts contained no salt, so I was losing salt without taking any in. Combined with heavy sweating, I was getting rid of sodium way too fast. I was only able to recover after I fully rehydrated and rested. No matter how healthy your diet is and how much water you're drinking, lack of sodium can lead to dehydration and even death if you don't catch it.

When you eat processed foods, most of the salt you eat is processed salt from those foods, as they are loaded with it. And by eating processed foods, you're also getting lots of preservatives, artificial colors, sugar, and so on, all of which can contribute to high blood pressure. But when you're eating an unprocessed diet, you don't have to worry about eating too much salt. The amount you are taking in won't be enough to cause water retention or other negative health effects. It's important to know that all salts are not created equal. For your cooking and sprinkling needs, skip table salt, which is a refined food, and choose unrefined sea salt or Himalayan salt, which are filled with minerals to nourish your body.

Staying properly hydrated keeps your spirits up and wards away anxiety and fatigue. It keeps you mentally alert because the brain requires hydration, too (it actually shrinks in volume when it's dehydrated). So, keep adding in the good by continuing to hydrate your plate!

TAKE A DEEP BREATH AND A BIG SIP

Before you make a bad food choice—the slice of cake from the office party, the comfort food candy, or the popcorn on the couch—take a deep breath. Stop, close your eyes for a moment, and think about your long-term goal. Is it enough to stop you from seeking short-term food satisfaction? Take a breath and reconnect with your driving core motivator (see page 25) and what you really want. Follow that with a glass of water and see whether it's worth it. If this doesn't do the trick, consider taking five minutes out to practice Diaphragm Breathing (page 259) so you can reconnect with the natural flow of your breath.

SWAP OUT
ONE GUILTY PLEASURE

I used to crave chocolate every day around three o'clock, and I wouldn't rest until I landed myself some. I wasn't even always hungry for it; it was just a habit. When I replaced the chocolate with a glass of lemon water, I was able to let go of the chocolate. I know, lemon water definitely doesn't taste like chocolate, but the point was to replace the habit and retrain my brain. Now I eat chocolate when I truly feel like it, in its superfood form—raw cacao powder or cacao nibs (read more about its benefits on page 117). One of my clients used to unwind and de-stress after work with a glass of wine. She replaced the wine with a quick workout followed by a hot bath. What's your go-to guilty pleasure? Replace it with something that's actually going to benefit you. It might not work immediately; keep at it until you've repeated it enough to make it a habit.

WHY WE FALL OFF TRACK

We set out with the best of intentions, but we can't get around the fact that we are human! Sometimes we fall off track, lose momentum, and suddenly we find ourselves polishing off a pint of ice cream. Why does this happen?

You may not be consciously aware of it, but there's a reward with every single action you take, even if it's a self-destructive action. The action of eating junk food might not take you in the direction of your goals, but you still get a reward: comfort. Until the pain of being uncomfortable outweighs the comfort this behavior brings, you'll continue to fall off track. What's the solution?

1. **Recognize what the reward is.** What secondary benefits are you getting? Revisit your vision board (page 13) and driving core motivator (page 25). If your DCM is not helping, then go back and revise it. Find something that sparks that emotion that reminds you why you're working toward your goals.

2. **Make the comfortable uncomfortable.** Leave your money in the car so you don't run to the snack machine at three o'clock. Keep the junk out of the house so you'll have to drive or walk to the store to get your fix.

3. **Cut down on TV if mindless eating is your binge-watch companion.** The reward is relaxation, but inevitably your willpower relaxes, too. Tell yourself you're going to have to do ten pushups or another vigorous exercise before you get to snack.

4. **Don't change into loose-fitting clothes as soon as you get home.** Keep your jeans or work clothes on and you'll be less likely to jump on the couch and snack on junk.

Step 9

Fill Your Plate with Anti-inflammatory Superfoods

To be worthy of the name *superfood*, a food must contain particularly high levels of phytonutrients, vitamins, minerals, and antioxidants, substances that can help protect our body from cell damage and prevent disease. Superfoods can be superfun: from tangy ferments to savory mushrooms, vegetables the color of the rainbow, chicken soup, and even chocolate. The following are ten of my favorites. I challenge you to eat from each group every day. They are a key component to aging in reverse! My ten-day meal plan will automatically pick them out for you, and from there you are invited to mix and match to make every meal a supermeal!

Dark Leafy Greens

Packed with fiber, vitamins, minerals, and antioxidants, dark leafy greens are an integral part of unprocessing your diet with absolutely no drawbacks. They're as close to that magic bullet for perfect health as you could possibly get!

Leafy greens can be a little bitter, which is a good thing: it reflects their high levels of calcium. As we age, we become more susceptible to osteoporosis, and green leafy vegetables can help retain the density of our bones. Their ample vitamin K partners up in supporting your bones.

Numerous studies have shown the cancer-fighting effects of leafy green vegetables, reflecting their high levels of antioxidants, carotenoids, flavonoids, and specific cancer-fighting compounds. Kale, collards, and mustard greens are part of the brassica family, which are known for their particularly powerful anticancer properties. The antioxidants and carotenoids in dark leafy greens help us with concentration and protect our brain from free radical damage. No one has ever complained of brain fog following a big green salad! In fact, research shows that people who eat green leafy vegetables daily have slower rates of cognitive decline as they age, making this superfood a veritable fountain of youth. You'll never feel overly full or go into a food coma from too many green vegetables, and the more consistent you are with your leafy greens, the more constant your energy levels will be.

Cabbage is also a nutritional powerhouse. My favorite way to eat it is fermented in the form of sauerkraut (page 174). To increase the chlorophyll content of cabbage to that of dark leafy greens, add a generous amount of dark green herbs, such as parsley, cilantro, or mint, to the mix.

MY GO-TO
DARK LEAFY GREENS

Arugula	Beet greens	Collard greens
Kale	Lettuce (the darker, the better)	Mustard greens
Spinach	Swiss chard	Turnip greens

If that all isn't enough, eating green leafy vegetables can boost your metabolism, which is strong incentive to keep consistent with your daily Super Salad (page 227)!

AN EASY ADD-IN

As leafy greens need little to no cooking, it takes little effort to supplement your dishes with a hit of them.

Stir chopped greens into stir-fries, stews, or chili.

Add a handful to your scramble.

Add greens to a soup or cup of bone broth (page 163).

Blend greens into smoothies.

Add a green garnish to any meal, including breakfast.

Sub greens for wraps or tacos (hearty collards and kale are great for this).

Brightly Colored Vegetables and Fruits

Eating the colors of the rainbow is a delicious way to plan your plate. And it's a surefire way to get in a variety of fruits and vegetables, each reflecting the various phytochemicals (a.k.a. phytonutrients) found in them. Phytonutrients are compounds produced by plants that give them their unique color, flavor, and smell. These compounds prevent them from threats from the environment, and by eating phytonutrient-rich vegetables, we protect ourselves from cell damage and disease. There are more than twenty-five thousand phytonutrients, so it's important to eat a wide range of colors to reap their various benefits.

RED FOODS contain large amounts of beta-carotene, the antioxidant quercetin, vitamins A and X, and lycopene, which has been shown to help protect against various forms of cancer. Red foods can help with heart health and ease in aging.

Red foods include: apples, cherries, cranberries, radishes, raspberries, red beets, red bell peppers, red-fleshed potatoes, red grapefruit, red onions, strawberries, tomatoes, and watermelon.

ORANGE FOODS also are high in the antioxidant beta-carotene, lycopene, and vitamins A and C. They support our eye and skin health, help lower blood pressure, and fight against arthritis and harmful free radicals in our body.

Orange foods include: apricots, butternut and other winter squash, cantaloupe, mangoes, nectarines, oranges, orange bell peppers, orange carrots, persimmons, pumpkin, sweet potatoes, and tangerines.

YELLOW FOODS contain the carotenoid zeaxanthin, a type of antioxidant connected with eye health. Compounds in yellow foods help protect from cancer and heart disease while strengthening the collagen in our skin. They are high in vitamin A, potassium, and lycopene.

Yellow foods include: bananas, corn, lemons, papaya, pineapple, pomelo, star fruit, yellow beets, yellow bell peppers, yellow grapefruit, and yellow pears.

GREEN FOODS are so powerful they've merited their own section!

In addition to the leafy greens listed on page 105, green foods include: artichokes, asparagus, broccoli, celery, green beans, okra, peas, and scallions.

BLUE/PURPLE FOODS look blue or purple from their phytochemicals called anthocyanins. They help protect against cardiovascular disease and support healthy aging. They contain resveratrol, known for its anti-aging properties.

Blue/purple foods include: blackberries, blueberries, eggplant, plums, purple (red) cabbage, purple carrots, purple-fleshed potatoes, and purple grapes.

AND DON'T OVERLOOK WHITE PRODUCE! The cholesterol- and blood pressure–lowering anthoxanthins, detoxifying sulfur, and anti-inflammatory properties of cauliflower, mushrooms (see pages 109 to 110), onions, garlic, and other light-hued vegetables and fruits are not to be missed.

Sea Vegetables

You might be thinking, *I'll pass on that superfood . . . there's no way I'm eating seaweed!* I have news for you: you already have. Seaweed is in foods you would never have considered: ice cream, baked goods, and bottled salad dressing, for example. But those are far from ideal sources of this superfood! Instead I'd like you to get adventurous and use sea vegetables in your daily cooking. If you need convincing, consider these amazing stats: vegetables from the sea typically have more overall nutrition than plants grown on land. Ounce for ounce, sea vegetables are higher in vitamins and minerals than *any other class of food*. Sea vegetables supply us all the minerals we need to live in proportions similar to our blood.

Benefits of sea vegetables include reducing cholesterol, removing radioactive elements from the body, softening tumors, and strengthening bones, teeth, and digestion. Seaweed helps us maintain healthy skin and hair. These are some of the more popular sea vegetable varieties:

DULSE is reddish brown with a salty, smoky flavor reminiscent of bacon. It can be found in whole leaf form to make a crunchy snack (page 231), and dulse flakes or powder can be added to or sprinkled over any number of dishes, from scrambled eggs to meatballs and chili.

ARAME is found in the form of dark brown to black stringlike strands and has a mild, sweet flavor. It pairs well with sweet vegetables, such as onions and carrots (see my recipe on page 203). Soak it in water before using to hydrate it.

WAKAME is a deep green or brown seaweed found in frond form and is most often served in salads and soups, such as the miso soup in Japanese restaurants. To use it, soak it in water to cover for twenty minutes, then drain and add it to a bowl of piping hot bone broth (page 163) or another soup.

KOMBU comes in dark brown strips or squares that are added to soups and stews to impart a savory flavor. I like to add a strip to bone broth.

BEFORE THERE WAS MSG

Before there was monosodium glutamate (MSG), there was seaweed. A substance called glutamic acid was isolated from kombu to make this chemical flavor enhancer. If you think a little MSG in your food isn't so bad, consider this: it can cause headaches, flushing, and neurological problems, and it has even been used to induce obesity in lab animals. Include sea vegetables in your cooking—a sprinkle of dulse, a scattering of wakame, or a strip of kombu tossed into your pot of bone broth (page 163)—for that natural savory flavor with no side effects other than off-the-charts nutrition!

NORI is most famous as a wrapper for sushi, and I love to wrap up all sorts of veggies with this sea vegetable (see page 243). Use it place of a flour wrap. The popular dried nori snacks are a deliciously addictive way to get in your sea veg.

* * *

Sea vegetables can be found in most natural food stores, increasingly in more mainstream supermarkets, and Asian markets. Look for convenient shakers of seaweed granules that you can sprinkle at the table.

Note: Sea vegetables are extremely high in iodine, an essential nutrient that regulates our thyroid. If you have a thyroid condition, check with your health-care provider before introducing sea vegetables into your diet.

Mushrooms

Whereas green vegetables contain chlorophyll and convert sunlight to food, mushrooms feed on dead matter. While that might not exactly sound appetizing, this demonstrates the ability of mushrooms to absorb and eliminate toxins and fight unwanted bacteria and viruses.

All mushrooms—from button to cremini and portobello—are natural detoxifiers. They're low in carbohydrates and calories and are a good source of B vitamins, trace minerals, and fiber. They are incredibly anti-inflammatory and have a high free radical–fighting antioxidant content. Studies have shown their strong anticancer properties, as they can help increase natural killer cells, immune cells that seek out and destroy cancerous cells. Mushrooms can slow down aging, stabilize blood sugar, and improve cardiovascular health. And as a bonus, mushrooms are a good source of glutamic acid, nature's version of MSG, adding a hit of savory flavor to any dish they are added to. Enjoy them in an omelet (page 189), soup, stir-fries, and even jerky (page 236).

Shiitake mushrooms are one of the healthiest foods you can put on your everyday shopping list. The compounds contained in shiitakes go the extra mile in the fight against inflammation, tumors, heart disease, and viruses, and they are unique for a plant in that they contain all eight essential amino acids. Maitake mushrooms, a.k.a. hen of the woods, are so powerful they are used as an adjunct treatment for cancer in Asia and can help minimize the effects of chemotherapy. Enjoy these as a treat, as they can be expensive and are not as widely available as other mushrooms (look for them in farmers' markets). Eat a variety of mushrooms to reap the benefits of each. Medicinal mushrooms to explore include reishi, cordyceps, chaga, lion's mane, and turkey tail. You might not have heard of these before, but they've been used in ancient medicine for *thousands* of years and can be highly beneficial to health. For example, cordyceps is a mushroom cousin linked to longevity, cancer prevention, blood sugar management, fat utilization, increased metabolism, heart health, and immune function. Chaga mushrooms are loaded with antioxidants, can help fight cancer, and can lower inflammation. Find these in liquid or capsule supplements at your natural food store.

Neglected Veggies

We've been taught to use just certain parts of our produce, and our landfills and compost piles are filled with lots of veggie waste. I consider the neglected parts of our produce superfoods because they deliver equal nutrition while extending your shopping dollar. Eating root to stem makes unprocessing your diet more affordable! Here are a few ideas to get you started:

Beet greens

Cook them as you would any other green.

Add to smoothies.

TIP: *Farmers' market shoppers often leave them behind, and they pile up. Ask farmers whether they have extra and they may give you a bunch for free. The same goes for turnip and radish leaves.*

Broccoli stems and leaves

Steam the leaves; they're just as nutritious as the florets.

Peel the stems and enjoy the crunchy insides as crudités, or thinly slice them and add them to stir-fries.

Blend into pesto.

Cabbage cores

Add them to your next batch of sauerkraut (page 174).

Carrot tops

Swap them into pesto for part of the basil.

Garlic, shallot, and onion tops and peels

Cook them with your bone broth (page 163; store them in the freezer until you have enough to make a batch).

Kale and collard stems

Juice them or add to smoothies.

Pickle them.

Finely chop them and cook them (they are tougher, so add them a few minutes before the leaves).

Lemon, lime, and orange peel

Zest them and add to flavor salad dressings, smoothies, and anywhere else you'd like a little added perk.

Throw the whole peels into water to make citrus water.

Mint stems

Chop them, put them in a teapot, and pour over boiling water. Steep for twenty minutes, then enjoy either hot or chilled as a no-cost mint tea. Or add them to bone broth (page 163) or Super Water (page 165).

Parsley and cilantro stems

Very finely chop them and add them to dishes along with the leaves.

Juice them or blend them into a smoothie.

Add them to a pot of bone broth (page 163).

Blend them into bone broth, strain, and enjoy a tasty green soup.

Make pesto out of them.

Scallion greens

Eat the whole scallion; the greens are every bit as tasty as the whites.

Chop the greens and use to top savory dishes and soups.

Strawberry tops

Make a digestive tea out of them by steeping in hot water for twenty minutes.

Add them to your Super Water (page 165) to infuse it with strawberry flavor.

Blend them along with the fruit into a smoothie.

Fermented Foods

From sauerkraut and kimchi to kombucha and yogurt, fermented foods offer probiotic gut and whole body-mind support. This superfood is so important I've dedicated a full section to it (see page 93). Eat ferments often!

Herbs and Spices

Spices add diversity to your food, transforming the same old into something special. And changing up your unprocessed plate is one of the most effective ways of staying on track with your diet. Herbs and spices have almost no calories, and they add antioxidant and anti-inflammatory superpowers to your food. Herbs count as vegetables, so think of herbs as way more than a garnish. Each has its own unique health benefits. Here are a few of my favorites:

BLACK PEPPER not only makes turmeric more bioavailable but works its same magic with most of our foods. Pepper is most flavorful and healthful when it's freshly ground; invest in a peppermill if you don't already have one.

CAYENNE adds more than just spice; its active ingredient, capsaicin, can clear congestion, relieve a headache, decrease pain, improve circulation, fight inflammation, help the body detox, and aid in weight loss. Studies have shown that people who eat spicy food tend to eat less of whatever is on their plate, as the capsaicin triggers the hunger satiety mechanism.

CILANTRO is both an herb and spice; the herb is cilantro, and the dried seeds are called coriander. Cilantro offers a fresh flavor (although some people avoid it, due to their having a genetic trait that makes it taste soapy) and a multitude of antioxidants, minerals, and vitamins to any food it's added to.

CINNAMON adds a sweet flavor but actually helps control blood sugar. It is good for digestion and soothing stomach issues. Its powerful polyphenols are cancer fighting and heart-healthy. Cinnamon has even been shown to fight tooth decay.

GINGER is an effective digestive aid and has cancer-inhibiting properties. It can relieve headaches, prevent colds, ease arthritis, and improve blood sugar levels. And its active ingredient, gingerol, has been found to burn body fat!

MINT is cooling, calming, and very high in antioxidants. It can help with digestion and can help relieve nausea and headache. Make a tea out of it or add it to salads, omelets, soups, and other dishes. If you love mint, plant a little in your yard and it will spread like crazy (or keep it in a pot if you want to contain it).

OREGANO has one of the highest antioxidant activity ratings of any food—more than forty times that of apples, for example. It is antifungal, antibacterial, anti-inflammatory, and anti-carcinogenic. A little fresh oregano adds a lot of flavor—try sprinkling some into scrambled eggs, salad dressing, and veggie dishes. And make sure to add a jar of dried to your pantry.

PARSLEY has a high fiber content and is an effective digestive aid, perhaps how it got its traditional place as a garnish on the plate (you're supposed to eat that garnish!). It's twice as high in iron as spinach and contains a good amount of vitamins A, C, and K.

ROSEMARY is a memory enhancer and helps to bring your mind into focus. It is also antibacterial and anti-inflammatory.

TURMERIC is one of nature's strongest anti-inflammatories and a spice I eat every day. It has a mild flavor, so a little won't change the flavor of your food (but too much will give it a bitter taste). Turmeric works best in conjunction with black pepper, so combine the two whenever you can. And sizzling turmeric in a little fat such as in a stir-fry makes it even more available to your body. Because inflammation is one of our greatest health concerns, I not only cook with turmeric, but supplement with it, too (see page 121).

Bone Broth

As several of my friends were turning fifty, I noticed they were looking noticeably fantastic, with smooth, vibrant skin and hardly a wrinkle. When I asked for their secret, the unanimous response was collagen. It wasn't a topical collagen beauty product, though. It was from consuming collagen in the form of bone broth. Bone broth is one of our oldest forms of nutrition, and it was making them look young! I needed no more convincing to start a bone broth habit.

Bone broth offers a delicious way for your body to take in collagen (though I like to supplement with collagen as well for extra protection; see page 120). Bone broth is easily digestible, and sipping on a cup of it will give you a boost while curbing your appetite. And it's just the thing for a cold, fever, or flu. A base of bone broth in place of water or packaged stock will up the flavor of soups, stews, and any other dish you add it to. It will instantly make you a better cook! Bone broth offers a multitude of nutritional benefits. Here are a few:

- Improves gut health

- Strengthens bones, muscles, and tendons

- Boosts immunity

- Fortifies hair and nails

- Reduces inflammation

- Reduces joint pain

- Curbs appetite

- Improves elasticity in skin

- Releases toxins

Thanks to its valuable collagen, vitamin, and mineral content, bone broth can reduce inflammation and thereby protect against many common health problems. I suggest enjoying bone broth every day, but it's up to you as to how much. You really can't overdo it. Making bone broth involves little more than adding bones and aromatics to a pot or slow cooker and simmering away. The hardest part is changing your mind-set to try something new! See my recipe on page 163 for how to do it. Or purchase packaged bone broth from your natural food store for convenience. Just look for the organic stuff, and if you make your own, use bones from organic meat.

Nuts, Seeds, and Coconut

Skip the chips to get your crunchy fix, because fiber-filled nuts and seeds are a snack that satisfies. I pack nuts and seeds into single-serving bags so I'll always have some on hand. I also make my own nut butter (page 169) and ferment a dairy-free cheese from nuts (page 170). Choose nuts and seeds in their unprocessed state, without added oil or salt.

Although nuts contain protein, they count as a fat when planning your plate (see pages 70 to 72). All nuts and seeds are a concentrated source of vitamins and minerals, in particular magnesium, zinc, calcium, and phosphorus. A few highlights: cashews contain tryptophan, which can reduce stress and relax you; pecans support the nervous system and heart; almonds are high in vitamin E and help regulate cholesterol and heart health; and walnuts, chia seeds, flaxseeds, and hemp seeds will wow you with their inflammation-busting omega-3 essential fatty acid content. Because our body can't make omega-3s, we need to consume them from food, and what better way than crunchy nuts and seeds! Read more about omega-3s on page 122. Note that peanuts are legumes, not nuts, and should be avoided.

Aim to eat a variety of nuts and seeds, both to please your palate and to make sure you're getting a variety of nutrients. For added incentive, studies show that people who eat nuts live longer and are less likely to get cancer or heart disease.

Coconut milk adds dairy-free creamy deliciousness to smoothies, soups, and desserts. So, don't fear the fat in coconut! It has high amounts of *healthy* fats in the form of medium-chain fatty acids. In particular, it contains lauric acid, which is easily absorbed by the body, used as energy, and helps burn fat. The fats in coconut can help improve heart health by lowering cholesterol and blood pressure. Dried coconut is another great way of getting this delicious superfood into your diet; sprinkle it onto a smoothie bowl, try it in my Almond Protein Bites (page 237), or add it to trail mix (page 238). Note that coconut milk in the can is the liquid extracted from coconut meat. Do not use cream of coconut, which is sweetened. The coconut beverage you'll find in the dairy case is often filled with sugar and stabilizers; choose an unsweetened version to add to coffee, tea, or smoothies.

Chocolate

If you're like 99.9 percent of people, you'll need no convincing to add this superfood to your plate! This food of the gods, dating back to ancient Mexico, doesn't need to be taken over by sugar to satisfy the chocoholic in you. But be careful, as the majority of chocolate we eat is in the form of milk chocolate candy, which contains very little cacao and mostly sugar. This is *not* the chocolate that scientific studies have given superfood status. For health benefits, raw cacao, the original source of chocolate, is the way to go. It's pure chocolate, bitter and rich tasting with no added sweetener. (Cocoa powder is roasted, which reduces the antioxidant content, but it is still a healthy choice.) A tablespoon of the powder contains fewer than 15 calories and will not stimulate insulin release. Cacao nibs, made from crushed cacao beans, are dried and fermented bits of cacao beans. Deep in pure chocolate flavor, they are slightly nutty and bitter tasting, like a grown-up chocolate chip!

What makes cacao a superfood? For one, it's one of the best sources of magnesium found in nature. Magnesium helps with sleep and healthy muscle and nerve function, and it keeps you regular (read more about magnesium on page 121). It is also high in potassium, phosphorus, copper, iron, manganese, and zinc. Cacao contains fiber, which helps you feel full, and it's super antioxidant rich. Chocolate can boost our mood because it contains compounds that increase levels of endorphins and serotonin in our brain. The same brain chemical—phenylethylamine—that is released when we experience feelings of love is found in chocolate. But you don't need to polish off a candy bar to cheer yourself up—when you swap in raw cacao for the processed stuff, you'll get that shot of bliss without the inevitable sugar crash that follows. Cacao can help stabilize blood sugar and reduce blood pressure, the risk of cardiovascular disease, cancer, and other chronic inflammatory conditions. The high polyphenol content—close to four hundred different compounds—of cacao can even boost cognitive function, making cacao a food that feeds your brain!

Stick to raw cacao powder or nibs for your daily chocolate enjoyment. Raw cacao can be enjoyed in smoothies (pages 190 and 195), protein balls (page 237), trail mix (page 238), and even chili (page 213)! For an occasional chocolate bar indulgence, choose one with a high cacao content—at least 70 percent—and low sugar. Stick to dark chocolate, as the dairy in milk chocolate can inhibit the absorption of chocolate's antioxidants, and keep your portions small.

DON'T GO DUTCH

Avoid cocoa powder labeled *Dutch-process* or *alkalized*. This means the powder has been processed with an alkalized solution, which makes it darker in color and milder. Since the bitter compounds in chocolate are the source of its phytochemicals and antioxidants, alkalization means most of those health-giving compounds are processed out. Stick to raw cacao to reap the benefits of this superfood.

Step 10

Supplement Your Plate

There are so many supplement choices, so many products, and sometimes less than knowledgeable salespeople telling you why you should buy something. The wrong information can not only put a very large dent in your pocketbook, but it can give you false hope and disappointment, and even make you sick. Over the years I have encountered so many bad supplements and wasted so much money on suggestions that I have become very untrusting of ads and endorsers promoting the latest and the greatest. However, I do believe supplements can have a place in health and healing. But first the bad news: there are no magic pills (other than V3; see page 75!). There's not a pill or drink that will make you leaner or stronger. That doesn't mean supplements can't enhance your health. What it does mean is that you can't eat a poor diet and be inactive and then pop a pill and get results. Without good nutrition and a healthy dose of exercise, results will not happen long term. The foundation is always going to be the Transformation Triangle: mind-set, an unprocessed plate, and a healthy weight. Supplements can *enhance* your efforts. Go to www.nataliejillfitness.com/resources to find my most current list of recommended brands. I keep this list updated as new information becomes available.

A REMINDER TO TAKE YOUR SUPPLEMENTS

Set out your supplements on your bedside the night before with a bottle of water alongside to prompt you to take them before starting your day. Supplement taking then becomes part of the mind-set task of Creating a Morning Routine (see page 33).

Collagen

Collagen plays an important role in skin, hair, nail, and bone health. So, in addition to enjoying bone broth (page 163), a rich source of collagen, I supplement with a collagen power for insurance and to replace what gets lost naturally through aging. There's even research showing that supplementing with collagen can lead to a noticeable reduction in skin dryness and wrinkles and an improvement in skin firmness. Collagen can also be beneficial for joint health and reduce joint pain.

Vitamin D

Vitamin D is affectionately known as the sunshine vitamin, because it's produced in your skin in response to sunlight. Few foods contain some vitamin D naturally; these include sardines, egg yolks, wild salmon, and shrimp. Many processed foods are fortified with vitamin D, but since you've unprocessed your diet, you won't be getting your D there.

Ten to fifteen minutes of real sun, not enough to tan or burn, whenever possible is the best way of getting vitamin D. But a vitamin D supplement will give you extra insurance. I take vitamin D, even though I live in sunny San Diego. That's because it's easy to fall deficient, which can cause us to lose focus and energy and leave us open to a number of health conditions. In fact, there's a vitamin D deficiency epidemic in this country.

Getting a sufficient amount of vitamin D is important for normal growth and development of bones and teeth as well as improved resistance against certain diseases including cancer, type 2 diabetes, chronic inflammation, and Alzheimer's disease. It also helps regulate the absorption of calcium and phosphorus and facilitates normal immune system function. Research has also shown that vitamin D might play an important role in regulating mood and warding off depression. Perhaps that's why we feel so good when we're out in the sun! Choose D_3, from animal sources, over D_2, from plant sources, as D_3 has been found to be much more effective in raising levels in the body.

Magnesium

Magnesium is the calming, antistress mineral that has the bonus effect of keeping inflammation down and keeping us regular. Sufficient magnesium reduces your risk for high blood pressure, and it has been shown to be extremely therapeutic when it comes to alleviating and preventing headaches, constipation, chronic pain, irritable bowel syndrome, and even asthma. Magnesium is found naturally in dark leafy greens, nuts, avocados, bananas, dark chocolate, and some dried fruits. It is also found in beans and whole grains. It is easy to fall short on magnesium in your diet, and it's especially important to supplement with magnesium when minimizing or eliminating beans and whole grains in your diet. I take magnesium in the evening, as it helps me relax and fall asleep. Topical magnesium can help with muscle aches and soreness.

Turmeric

I mentioned turmeric earlier and I'll mention it again here; it has so many healing properties that I not only cook with it liberally, but I supplement with it, too. Turmeric is one of nature's most potent anti-inflammatories and may relieve arthritis and digestive complaints and prevent cancer. In fact, a number of studies have even reported that using curcumin, the active ingredient in turmeric, can help more than certain prescriptions. India, where turmeric is enjoyed daily, has one of the world's lowest rates of Alzheimer's disease. Look for a supplement that also contains black pepper, as the pepper enables to turmeric to be better absorbed into your bloodstream.

Fish Oil

Fish oil, from the tissues of oily fish, is an important source of omega-3 fatty acids, which are crucial for joint health, keeping inflammation at bay, and all bodily functions. One study showed that omega-3 fish oil supplements worked just as well as NSAIDs in reducing arthritic pain and are a safer alternative to NSAIDs, known to create stomach problems and bleeding.

There's no one-size-fits-all recommendation for omega-3s, as your needs will vary depending on your health, age, and diet, and if you're eating fish regularly, you may not need to supplement. But I highly suggest taking an omega-3 supplement in addition to what you get in food for insurance purposes. This is because according to research conducted at Harvard University, omega-3 fatty acid deficiency is, shockingly, one of the top ten causes of death in America. This is totally preventable! A general guideline is somewhere between 250 to 500 milligrams of EPA and DHA for the standard, healthy adult. And when it comes to choosing a brand of fish oil, quality trumps quantity, so try to steer clear of cheap, big-box store versions and spend your money on higher-quality options that will deliver a product your body can make better use of. There are many lists online of top-rated brands and capsules, so do your research. Once you open the bottle, keep it in the fridge to extend its shelf life. Note: There's no need to supplement with omega-6s (see sidebar).

Telomere Support

Telomeres are segments of our DNA at the end of our chromosomes. As we age, more of our cells lose their telomeres and the body follows and begins breaking down. Their shortening process has been linked with aging, cancer, and a higher risk of death. Although telomere shortening related to age is inevitable, there are things we can do to help slow the loss of or restore telomere length. We can reduce stress, lose excess fat, stay active, and eat an unprocessed diet. And there are some promising supplements to help. I take and recommend a telomere support supplement daily for this.

WHEN SUPPLEMENTING, STICK TO OMEGA-3 AND SKIP OMEGA-6

As you have learned, not all fats are bad, and in fact, fatty acids benefit our body quite literally in every way imaginable, boosting the health of our skin, respiratory system, brain, all vital organs, and circulatory system.

The fats we get from omega-3 and omega-6 fatty acids are key to an overall functioning and healthy body, including reducing inflammation, increasing focus, and aiding in weight loss and heart health. We need both to live, but our body does not produce them on its own. Instead, to get them, we have to seek them out from the food we eat or in supplement form.

Sources of omega-3s include seafood (e.g., sardines, salmon, tuna, and herring), certain grains, walnuts, hemp seeds, flaxseeds, chia seeds, pumpkin seeds, Brazil nuts, and spirulina. Omega-6s are abundant in foods, and in fact, our modern diets are feeding us way more of them than we actually need, largely from processed vegetable oils. The ideal ratio is two to one omega-3s to omega-6s, meaning you should be getting double the omega 3s to hit the ideal daily dosage. However, thanks to the frozen foods, fast-food meals, and high-calorie, high-sugar, and high-sodium foods that grace most of our grocery store shelves, the opposite is actually becoming a reality for many of us. In fact, it has been found that many people are getting up to twenty times more omega-6s than omega-3s.

Since you have started unprocessing your diet, you are likely consuming less of the unhealthy sources of omega-6s, but you may still be getting them in such foods as sunflower oil, safflower oil, or sesame oil, nuts, seeds, grains, and leafy green veggies, such as kale and broccoli. This is important to be aware of because excessive amounts of omega-6s can contribute to inflammation and result in heart disease, cancer, asthma, arthritis, and depression. Since we need omega-6s for healthy function of our cells, we don't want to eliminate them altogether. Just be aware of your ratios, supplement with omega-3 in the form of fish oil, and skip the omega-6 supplements.

Branched-Chain Amino Acids (BCAAs)

The double-edged sword of dieting is that you reduce your caloric intake to lose weight and lean out, but the leaner your body gets, the harder it works to hold on to fat stores, which means it can lead to muscle breakdown. Your body would rather tap into existing muscle than fat for energy! With less lean muscle mass, your metabolism will slow down. Branched-chain amino acids to the rescue! BCAAs are known to increase protein synthesis and decrease muscle protein breakdown while reducing muscle soreness after workouts. This supplement is great for postworkout recovery, preventing fatigue, and gaining or preserving muscle mass and preventing fatigue.

Probiotics

Probiotics boost our body's ability to absorb nutrients and fight infections. They support immune function and healthy digestion as well as beautiful skin. Historically, we had plenty of probiotics in our diet from eating fresh foods from good soil and by fermenting our foods to keep them from spoiling. However, because of modern agricultural practices, our food contains little to no probiotics today, and even worse, many foods actually contain dangerous antibiotics that kill off the good bacteria in our body. So, by adding more probiotic foods and a supplement to your diet, you will strengthen your immune system. See page 93 to learn about the probiotic benefits of eating fermented foods.

Greens Powder

You know who you are . . . if you have a hard time eating your greens or getting enough in each day, a good greens powder is key. Concentrated greens superfood means you're getting mega phytonutrients and lots of veggies in one serving. The benefits range from boosting your energy levels to helping digestion, purifying your body, and enhancing your immune system. Choose a powder without added sweeteners (a little stevia is okay) and artificial colors or flavors. And remember, this doesn't take the place of eating your veggies, but does act as an insurance policy for getting your greens.

HERBAL REMEDIES FOR OUR HORMONES

Nature provides us with powerful medicine to ease hormonal symptoms. Ginseng has long been used in alternative medicine to boost energy and generally improve vitality and emotional balance. Lemon balm and passionflower have both been found to ease crankiness and nervousness and naturally lull you into a more balanced, calm state. Maca has shown promising research results as a remedy in perimenopausal women, and dandelion and milk thistle may also help relieve symptoms of menopause. With no harmful side effects (make sure you consult your doctor if you're on any medications), you can take these remedies before bed and they'll also help improve your sleep, minimizing symptoms of brain fog, irritability, and fatigue.

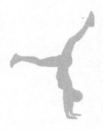

Step 11

What Changing Hormones Bring to Your Plate (What the Heck Is Going On?)

If you're a woman, the words *perimenopause* and *menopause* probably elicit some type of strong feeling from you. Maybe they bring up such emotions as nervousness, uncertainty, dread, or confusion. Perhaps you're currently in the throes of perimenopause or menopause. It's a crucial time in any woman's life, so whether you've not yet approached these changes, are in the thick of it, or the time is behind you, understanding perimenopause and menopause is crucial for you.

Perimenopause is the phase leading up to menopause; it simply refers to the gradual process that transitions your body from regularly ovulating and having a period to no longer doing either. It's different from premenopause, which is the time before perimenopause when you still have regular periods. During perimenopause, which typically lasts about four years but can extend anywhere from a few months to as long as ten years, you'll start to have an irregular period and possibly other uncomfortable symptoms (read on for more about those). **Menopause** is the natural end to menstruation and is technically hit when a woman hasn't menstruated in twelve months.

When our body enters perimenopause, usually in our forties but sometimes sooner or later, production of hormones begins to change, and this is when the symptoms of menopause begin to kick in. Levels of estrogen, which is the main female hormone in the body, begin to steadily decline. By the time we reach menopause, we're producing so little estrogen that our periods stop altogether. To a lesser extent, the female hormone progesterone and the male hormone testosterone, both present in our body, also begin to drop. As a trifecta, the changing levels of all three of these can have myriad effects on our mood, sex drive, energy, anxiety levels, and more. Including of course, our weight.

The Perfect Storm for Weight Gain

You've likely all heard of the common-suspect symptoms associated with hormone changes, whether or not you've personally gone through them yourself yet. Mood swings, hot flashes (I've definitely experienced these!), bone loss, and changes in hair and skin. And if you're like many women, you might be wondering what it will do to your waistline. Here's the gist of what to expect, and what you can do to continue feeling your best.

You've no doubt heard or experienced by now how any fluctuation in hormones can spell chaos for your weight, whether a result of a condition, such as thyroid disease; from taking certain medications; or because of natural changes such as menopause. It's true; any change in hormones can certainly throw off the delicate balance of your body. So, you're right to wonder what menopause means in terms of the number you see on the scale or the image that looks back at you in the mirror.

Although there's no scientific evidence that menopause itself is solely responsible for weight gain—aging itself plays a role in gaining weight—the changes that our body experiences during this transition can be a major contributing factor. The lowering of estrogen hormone levels makes aging even more complex for women than men. Estrogen plays a direct role in moderating our weight, our metabolism, our appetite, and the way we store fat. A drop in estrogen in an aging body is the perfect storm for gaining weight!

During menopause, the body's metabolism naturally slows down. Part of this has to do with aging—older bodies naturally use less energy and require fewer calories—but part of this is a side effect of menopause. A slowed metabolism means your body burns fewer calories each day, and this will lead to weight gain if you continue eating the same amount of food. To make matters worse, estrogen also helps control levels of compounds that stimulate appetite, so when estrogen levels drop, levels of these compounds increase and so do your appetite, which can lead to overeating—the last thing you need when your metabolism slows down!

SOME RELATED REASONS FOR WEIGHT GAIN

Metabolism and Body Temperature

One reason why we gain weight during menopause has to do with a slight drop in body temperature. Between 40 and 80 percent of a person's energy expenditure is used to maintain core body temperature, so even a small decrease in body temperature can mean a huge decrease in metabolism, which can ultimately lead to weight gain. One study found postmenopausal women were on average 0.25°C cooler than premenopausal women. This equates to a 3.25 percent drop in energy expenditure, which is 65 fewer calories burned every day. For a typical fifty-year-old postmenopausal woman who is 150 pounds and 5 foot 4, this would lead to gaining 6.7 pounds in a year just because of temperature!

Sleep Deprivation and Weight Gain

Low estrogen and shifting hormone levels during menopause can make it tough for women to get enough quality sleep, and disrupted sleep is directly linked to weight gain. A large study found women who slept five hours or less gained more weight than women who clocked more than seven hours every night. One of the reasons this can happen is because it's tougher to follow healthy lifestyle behaviors, such as eating nutritious food and exercising, when you're chronically fatigued.

And it doesn't stop there. During perimenopause and menopause, it's natural for your lean body mass to start decreasing and body fat to start accumulating. Decreases in estrogen and progesterone actually change the way fat is metabolized and stored, increasing the rate of fat storage and decreasing a woman's ability to burn fat. In addition to storing fat at a faster rate, the places where fat is stored start to change, too. As you may have noticed, that fat buildup can shift from the thighs and hips into the abdominal area, the most dangerous place to gain weight, thanks to hormonal changes. Abdominal fat is metabolically active and secretes such substances as adipokines.

Adipokines act as hormones that talk to organs including the brain, immune system, liver, muscle, and the adipose tissue it comes from, and they also regulate inflammation. An overload of adipokines is a trigger for inflammation and is linked to obesity, type 2 diabetes, heart disease, and other health complications.

Other Ways Changing Hormones May Affect You
Brain Fog

You've probably heard of (or experienced) the "brain fog" that comes along with menopause. Turns out, this isn't a myth, and memory issues can be completely normal during menopause. Hormones, particularly a hormone called estradiol (it's in the estrogen family), influence parts of the brain that support memory. As levels of estrogen hormones drop during perimenopause and menopause, the brain undergoes changes, too, and this is where mild brain fog can come in. Eating an unprocessed diet, especially foods high in omega-3 fatty acids, exercising regularly, getting enough sleep, and keeping your brain active (think: reading and doing puzzles) can help reduce the menopausal brain fog.

Why Am I So Tired?

Along with brain fog, if you've reached or gone through perimenopause or menopause, you know it can feel like a never-ending afternoon slump. Nearly 90 percent of menopausal women feel fatigue several times per week, and this has a lot to do with hormonal changes. Hormones are responsible for regulating energy levels, and they're also involved in sleep. When hormone levels drop, so does your energy, and irregular sleep patterns can contribute to fatigue, too. What can you do to counteract this? Eat an unprocessed diet, drink plenty of water, be active every day, start a meditation or mindfulness practice (see page 39 for mine), and practice proper sleep hygiene by banishing electronics from the bedroom, investing in a quality mattress and sheets, avoiding eating close to bedtime, and keeping the thermostat low at night.

The Bone Connection

As if brain fog and exhaustion aren't enough, as we age, bone density becomes more and more of a concern, especially in menopausal women. Estrogen helps regulate bone density, and when we lose estrogen during menopause, the risk for osteoporosis and fractures goes up. You can help reduce your risk by eating foods that contain calcium, vitamin D, and protein; limiting alcohol; and by doing strength-training exercises. Consuming probiotics can also support your bones because they've been shown to inhibit production of osteoclasts, which are cells that break down bone and contribute to bone loss and osteoporosis.

How to Look and Feel Your Best

You may ask, "How will perimenopause and menopause and the changing hormones associated with them ultimately end up affecting my health, the way I feel, and the way I look?" And of course, "What can I do about it?"

First, don't forget about mind-set (see Part 1 on page 11)! Don't believe self-imposed stops that hormonal changes will inevitably slow you down, age you, and pack on the pounds. When you reset your thinking, food becomes the most powerful tool in the medicine cabinet for easing away unwanted mood swings, sugar cravings, and bloat and for managing your weight. What you put on your plate is the most important factor in managing your weight and your first line of defense against the symptoms associated with peri-menopause and menopause. Here are some guidelines.

Amp Up the Protein

During menopause, it's natural for our body to start losing muscle, so it's up to us to overcome this through diet and exercise. Research shows eating 25 to 30 grams of protein at each meal can help maintain muscle mass, so now's the time to really amp up the protein.

Protein (along with exercise) builds lean muscle, which keeps our metabolism at optimum function, just what we need to stabilize our hormones when they're in flux. A steady metabolism can also help with weight management because we burn calories throughout the day. Protein is also key for keeping our bones healthy and strong and our hair, nails, and skin looking their best.

Most people do a good job getting in enough protein at dinner, but you need to make sure you're eating protein all throughout the day. Unfortunately, the reality is most women actually start to eat less protein at this time in life, which significantly increases risk for weight gain. The meal plan (see page 158) will help you get enough protein into every meal of the day.

Go Organic

I recommend that everyone choose organic foods as often as possible, but going organic becomes more important during menopause to help reduce our exposure added hormones, along with pesticides and GMOs.

When it comes to meat and dairy, if you decide to reintroduce it, this is especially important. Conventionally raised cows are usually given hormones to speed up growth or regulate reproduction, and these hormones get into the meat and milk (and onto your plate). During menopause, the last thing you need is an influx of outside hormones when you're struggling to get a handle on your own. Hormones are prohibited in organic farming, so choosing organic meat and dairy is a must. Chickens are never given hormones, but they are often given antibiotics if they aren't organic, and you want to avoid those, too.

Eat Your Ferments

There couldn't be a better time to start a fermentation habit (see page 93) or take a probiotic supplement (see page 124) than now, as when we have a bacterial imbalance in the gut (which the majority of people do), it can interfere with how our hormones are acting.

Imbalanced hormones can increase risk of high blood pressure, so menopausal women are certainly vulnerable, and there's tons of evidence showing probiotics can lower this risk. Taking probiotics can also promote bone health and help prevent osteoporosis (which we know is a big concern right now), decrease menopause symptoms, reduce inflammation, and lessen stomach discomfort.

Bacteria in the gut isn't the only thing that changes during menopause. The microbiome of our lady parts is altered, too, thanks to decreasing levels of estrogen, and taking probiotics can help restore the balance down there. Urinary tract infections are another common issue postmenopausal women face, and probiotics can help prevent these from happening.

Be Strict About Sugar

We all know we should avoid it (read more on page 79), yet it's all too easy to fall back. As soon as you have some, you'll want more, and with hormone changes, it's going to get even harder. For menopausal women, sugar can add fuel to the fire and irritate already undesirable symptoms, such as mood swings, bone loss, and hot flashes. Think of sugar as a trigger for everything you don't want when it comes to menopause. It impacts how the body metabolizes estrogen, and estrogen is the catalyst for weight gain.

Menopause affects the body's ability to process blood sugar. Women who reduce or eliminate sugar during this time will likely lose the most weight and keep it off long term. Since I have told you to watch your intake of all things sugar, it wouldn't be farfetched to assume that maybe going the artificial route will be your best bet, but in reality this can present an even bigger problem. A number of studies have found artificial sweeteners kick hormonal issues into high gear. This is the last thing you want when your hormones are already changing. Whether you are menopausal or not, artificial sweeteners have been linked to higher rates of diabetes and metabolic syndrome, not to mention old-fashioned weight gain. Read more about the fake sweet stuff on page 84.

Make Produce Your First Choice for Carbs

Whenever possible, make vegetables (excluding potatoes and corn) and fruits your first choice for carbs. Although it can be tempting to fall prey to dietary advice telling you to ditch the carbs altogether, reaching for fruits, veggies, and the unprocessed choices and combining them with good fats and proteins all will keep your blood sugar levels constant and energy levels up.

What About Soy?

Soy is a hot-button topic in the dietary community. Does it alleviate menopause symptoms, or should you avoid it? There's a ton of mixed information about soy out there, especially when it comes to hormones and cancer prevention, so what's the deal? Turns out, the studies that show soy may be beneficial are from countries where soy is a staple in the diet, so the people have eaten soy throughout their entire lives. In the United States, where most soy is genetically modified, heavily processed, and found in such forms as soy protein isolate and not introduced until later in life, that beneficial effect does a complete 180 and soy becomes harmful to health. Some health-care professionals recommend soy as a remedy for mood swings and hot flashes because it naturally contains high amounts of the phytoestrogen isoflavones, which mimics the effects of estrogen in the body. If you truly know that you have low estrogen levels, it may make sense to add some soy in after you've finished the plan, but you'd want to confirm that first. If you do try soy, make sure it's non-GMO and organic.

Make Food Your First Line of Defense

While stocking up your grocery cart, remember to keep in mind all the commonsense healthy eating wisdom you've been learning throughout the book. Food is a natural and delicious means of easing away unwanted mood swings, sugar cravings, and bloat. Eat your Daily Super Salad (page 227) to get in those all-important greens and enjoy a selection of superfoods (see pages 104 to 118) daily. Stay clear of inflammation triggers, eat the colors of the rainbow, sip on bone broth, enjoy raw cacao, and make food your medicine. With the mouthwatering recipes that follow, that won't be hard to accomplish!

Step 12

Next Steps

This book builds on the mission of my previous book, *7-Day Jump Start*—unprocessing your diet—and takes it up a notch to reset your body to meet its changing needs. You've added more volume to your veggies, you've boosted your diet with daily superfoods, and you've removed all sweeteners except for fruit. You've also given your body a break from dairy, grains, beans (including soy), and legumes, as these can be hard to digest and a source of inflammation. Removing them from my diet was a big part of my comeback from the inflammation and weight gain that came with a severe injury.

It's important to stick as close to the plan as possible for the full ten days, or until you've reached your health and fat-loss goals. At that point, you'll likely feel so fantastic that you'll want to keep going, and I invite you to do so if you wish. But if you would like to try adding foods back, incorporate them one a time and see how you feel. There's no scientific way to do it, but one food a week is a safe way to go. If you add everything at once and you don't feel great, you won't know the culprit and you'll have to start over again. For example, if you want to add dairy, you could have a plain organic Greek yogurt for breakfast on Monday, then if you're feeling great by the end of the week, consider adding moderate amounts of dairy the following week and then introduce another food, such as small portions of gluten-free grains, and see how you feel. Continue to avoid refined sugar and artificial sweeteners and use fruit as your main sweetener. With the amazing fruit-sweetened desserts I'm sharing with you, including fudge (page 240) and cheesecake (page 241), I promise you won't feel deprived!

Adding Back Dairy

If you decide to reintroduce dairy, going organic is especially important. Conventionally raised cows are usually given hormones to speed up growth or regulate reproduction, and these hormones get into the meat and milk (and onto your plate). As mentioned in the previous chapter, during menopause, the last thing you need is an influx of outside hormones when you're struggling to get a handle on your own. Hormones are prohibited in organic farming, so choosing organic dairy is a must.

Start with a fermented dairy, such as yogurt or kefir, preferably organic and made from raw milk dairy if possible. If you do well with these, try other dairy products, such as cheese, but always keep it organic.

If you're someone who likes to supplement with whey protein powder, you may try adding it back in at this time.

Sample serving sizes:

- ½ cup plain Greek yogurt or cottage cheese (counts as a protein)

- 1½ tablespoons cheese (counts as a fat)

Adding Back Grains and Legumes

First, remember that I do not recommend adding gluten—wheat, barley, and rye—back to your diet at all. Add grains and legumes one at a time, leaving at least three days in between each new food, and see how you react. To make them more digestible, soak them in water to cover for a few hours or overnight and discard the water before cooking to remove the antinutrients they contain that can impede digestion (read more about these on page 88). Because white rice does not contain an outer layer of bran, it does not require soaking and is more digestible for some people.

One more trick is to try cooling your grains to make them starch resistant. Resistant starch, as the name implies, is starch that resists digestion. This means it is not digested in the stomach or small intestine and reaches the colon intact. The starch thus acts like soluble fiber and feeds friendly bacteria, improving digestion and having a positive effect on blood sugar. All that's needed to make grains and legumes starch resistant is to cool them to 130°F or below after cooking.

Sample serving sizes (counts as a starchy carb):

- ½ cup cooked white rice

- ½ cup cooked brown rice

- ½ cup cooked quinoa

- ½ cup cooked millet

- ½ cup cooked gluten-free pasta

- ½ cup cooked oatmeal

- ½ cup cooked chickpeas or other beans

- 1 (6-inch) 100 percent corn tortilla

The 95 Percent Rule

In the reality of life, it's what you do 95 percent of the time that matters. I'll never tell you that you can never eat a processed food again. The world won't come to an end. No food is off limits forever unless it causes a strong reaction when you eat it. If you start feeling off or are putting on weight, it's time to dial it back, consider taking a longer break from the foods in question, or repeat the plan for another ten days. As you enjoy newfound confidence in your body and your daily food choices, you'll no longer have to measure portions precisely because your body will know when it's hungry and when it's full. It will know exactly what it needs. How empowering is that!

Keeping It Up

While this is a ten-day plan, to take it to the next level, I recommend keeping it up for a full month to get the full taste of it. As you reach your weight- and fat-loss goals, you will be able to increase your portions. In fact, you won't have to watch portions anymore because you'll know just when you're hungry and when you've had enough.

Many of my clients say they feel so good they don't want to go back to how they ate before, and they just keep going. Without grains and dairy in their diet, they don't feel the effects of inflammation and they get the full benefits of aging in reverse. It becomes more than a plan but a lifestyle, and they just don't feel their best when they go back to how they used to eat. Think of it this way: if you walk by a polluted river and you throw in a piece of trash, you won't really notice. But if you clean up that river and then toss in some garbage, it will be obvious. You wouldn't throw trash into a river anyway, so it makes sense that you would treat your body with the same respect!

....
Transformation
....

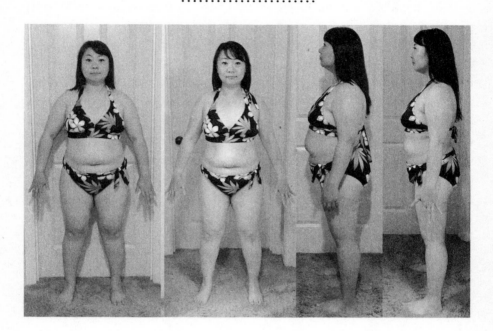

YULANDA

"I Fell in Love with Eating Real Food"

Before working with Natalie, I had suffered from depression for many years. I felt people would see my weight, not the real me. I come from a Chinese background where food is more than just fuel for the body but an expression of love. My family, not known for being subtle, thought they were doing me a service by telling me I needed to lose weight, but they themselves weren't in the greatest shape. I was so confused about nutrition.

I tried a number of diets, cleanses, pills, and food bars, all of which didn't work, and I would always gain the weight back and then some. This was my life's cycle, so when I found Natalie Jill's program, I doubted whether I could do it or even understand it. To my happy surprise, the work went beyond food and exercise and into mind-set. I'd never seen or heard other programs talk about mental state, and this is what got me through the program and helped me sustain the changes I'd made. I created a vision board by honing in on where I wanted to go and what kind of person I wanted to be. I cut out pictures of places where I wanted to live and how I wanted to live my life, beyond food and being skinny. My goal was to be free, to break away from the bondage of being a perfectionist. My self-imposed stop was "I can't do it." I was all or nothing because I was afraid of failing. I replaced that self-imposed stop with making a decision to focus on what I *can* do and finish the program no matter what. And I wound up losing 24 pounds!

Growing up, I never developed a taste for veggies and fruits, but I've always loved food. My friends called me a "foodie," and I used to eat out just about every meal. All my social media revolved around food. Being a foodie was the only thing I could be proud of. Without it, I felt like I was nothing. But I decided to make a commitment to cook for myself as a first step to unprocessing my diet. At first, just being in the kitchen was intimidating. I didn't even know where the salt was! So, I stuck to basics: I made sure to get a balance of carbs, protein, and fat in every meal. I told myself I'd just put my "foodie" label on hold for six weeks. But then everything changed when I discovered how good I felt with this way of eating! I started to be less fearful of the kitchen. I reset my palate and even veggies started to taste good. I was satisfied with what I put on my plate. Then when I'd eat a little of what I used to eat, I'd feel greasy, bloated, and thirsty. I'd go into a food coma and would need a nap. So now, I don't make exceptions for special occasions because I just don't want to feel that way anymore.

Eating an unprocessed diet energizes me, and for the first time in my life, I can really taste my food without the extra fat and fillers that disguised their original flavor. No wonder I thought I didn't like real food! Once I reset my diet, I decided I could still call myself a foodie—an unprocessed foodie! I was so inspired I started an Instagram page to share the photos of the clean food I now enjoy to remind me of my favorites, keep myself motivated, and inspire friends to eat this way.

Step 13

Planning to Plan Your Plate: Everything You Need for Easy Meal Planning

Get ready for ten days of incredible unprocessed meals! The focus of the meal plan will keep you on track and committed to following through. I've provided plenty of swap outs for variety and flexibility, but if formal recipes aren't your thing, you can easily build your own meals using the formula on page 152.

Keep in mind that meal prep is a lot easier when you take the time to think ahead. To the best of your ability, have ingredients on hand and schedule time on your calendar. Now, let's set your kitchen and mind-set up for success! To start, let's fill your fridge and pantry.

Unprocess Your Shopping List

With endless choices to tempt, taunt, and confuse us, a trip to the grocery store can quickly put us into a state of overwhelm. But with your unprocessed grocery list in hand, navigation becomes easier and makes shopping more efficient. That's because charting your course is easier when you get to bypass the aisles filled with junk—which is most of them! Here's how to start:

1. **Stay outside.** Shop the perimeters of the store. This is the easiest way to make sure you're getting unprocessed foods. There you'll find produce, meat, eggs, and fermented foods. The few things you'll pick out in the inner aisles include oils, vinegars, coconut milk, canned tomatoes, nuts, grain-free crackers, and, if you go back to eating them, grains and legumes. Almost everything else is processed.

2. **Think rainbow.** Make your basket colorful. This ensures that your food is full of variety. Red, orange, yellow, purple, green—every color that exists in nature and makes up an unprocessed diet. Unless it's pumped up with artificial food coloring, most processed food is similar in color, generally a shade of brown, tan, or white.

3. **Pay attention to labels.** The devil is in the details. Get hyperfocused here! Is there no label? Then, it's natural! Celery? Apple? Banana? You get it. But if there is a label, read the ingredients. Don't just look at calorie, carb, and sugar count. How many ingredients are in it? Do you know what all of the ingredients are? Fewer is generally better.

4. **Check the shelf life.** If it lasts a long time, it's likely processed or preserved, perhaps containing hydrogenated oils and fillers, and you should steer clear of it. The shorter the shelf life, the longer the potential for your life.

5. **Prioritize organic and non-GMO.** Make sure that you are making the best choices for your health that fit into your budget. As I mentioned earlier, the Environmental Working Group (ewg.org) keeps an updated "Dirty Dozen" list of the most highly sprayed produce. Prioritize going organic with those fruits and veggies.

6. **Take healthy shortcuts.** Choose timesaving options, such as prewashed lettuce and spinach, fresh fruit bowls, prechopped vegetables, and riced cauliflower. It's not cheating if it gets you to eat your veggies!

7. **Plan.** Before you go, make a thorough list so you are sure of what you are picking up. Ideally, go to the store twice a week to get the freshest foods, but if that doesn't work for your schedule, buy in bulk and

freeze. If you have a local farmers' market, try to plan trips there for fresh, seasonal produce. And never go to the store hungry. You will definitely go home with more than you need!

Fill Your Pantry

The following list contains everything you'll need for the ten-day meal plan and beyond. Supplement with your protein, produce, and perishable choices from the lists on pages 154 to 156 and from the individual recipes and you're ready to cook.

Oils and Vinegars

Extra-virgin olive oil

Virgin (unrefined) coconut oil

Toasted sesame oil

Cider vinegar

White wine vinegar

Condiments and Packaged Goods

Boxed bone broth (if not making your own; make sure it is organic)

Hot sauce

Dijon mustard (check label to be sure it's gluten-free)

Capers

Asian fish sauce

Coconut aminos (a soy-free soy sauce substitute made from coconut)

Coconut milk (canned pure)

Coconut cream (not cream of coconut, just pure coconut)

Water-packed tuna

Tomato sauce (no-sugar-added)

Tomato paste

Canned diced tomatoes

Sea Vegetables

Arame

Dulse granules

Dulse leaf (whole)

Nori

Wakame

Nuts, Seeds, and Coconut

Raw whole almonds

Slivered almonds

Raw cashews

Raw pecans

Raw walnuts

(Continues)

(Nuts, Seeds, and Coconut Continued)

Unsweetened almond or other nut milk (if not making your own)

Unsweetened almond or other nut butter (if not making your own)

Tahini (sesame paste)

Unsweetened coconut flakes

Unsweetened shredded coconut

Cacao nibs

Chia seeds

Sesame seeds

Poppy seeds

Pumpkin seeds

Baking Ingredients

Almond flour

Baking powder

Baking soda

Raw cacao powder

Pure almond extract

Pure vanilla extract

Dried fruit

Currants

Dried dates

Dried figs

Goji berries

Raisins

Herbs and Spices

Caraway seeds

Cayenne pepper

Celery seeds

Chili powder

Chipotle chile powder

Dried oregano

Dried sage

Dried thyme

Garlic powder

Ground allspice

Ground cinnamon

Ground cumin

Ground turmeric

Nutmeg

Onion powder

Paprika

Red pepper flakes

Sea salt or Himalayan salt

Whole black peppercorns

Supplements

Protein powder

Greens powder

Set Your Fridge Up Like a Salad Bar

As soon as you get home from the grocery store or farmers' market, *before* you put anything away, make it as user-friendly and quick to get at as possible. Think: salad bar fridge! This step is key to following through with your commitment to healthy eating, in particular V3 (see page 75). I want to get you out of the habit of leaving your produce in the bag, throwing it in the fridge, and losing it to the bottom of the crisper drawer. Not only is it more likely to go bad, but you're less likely to grab it because you've forgotten all about it. With all the veggies I want you to get into your plate, this is key! Here's what I do:

- Unpack and immediately clean off the vegetables and fruit, and dry them.
- Chop the veggies and separate them into single-use resealable plastic bags or clear glass containers so you can easily start a sauté, add V3 to an omelet, or complete a soup.
- Put whole fruit in glass bowls so it looks inviting, not only to you but your whole family.
- Prep salad greens and keep them in bowls or to-go containers ready to be tossed with dressing.
- Put your herbs in a vase with water. They'll keep longer and make an edible bouquet.
- Precook proteins, such as chicken and turkey, so you can quickly add them to salads or complete a main dish. Even opening a can of tuna and transferring it to a container can make or break your decision to bring lunch to the office or whip up a salad for dinner rather than grabbing junk or going to a restaurant.
- Hard- or soft-boil your eggs. Put them right into your fridge's egg holders.
- Put nuts into individual snack bags.
- Invest in silicone suction lids. This eliminates the need to put food into containers and saves on washing up and using plastic wrap. They're also great for leftovers—just pop the lid on and stick it in the fridge.

I know this sounds like a ton of prep; but trust me, it's worth it—you'll be surprised how a few hours just one day a week can make meals a snap, whether you're packing a lunch or planning dinner.

Have a Go-to List for Travel

Being away from home can be tricky, which is why it pays to be prepared. Here's what I keep on hand to put into my unprocessed foods travel kit. It's reassuring to know that a good source of protein and fat is always in reach!

- Nuts and seeds
- Grain-free crackers
- Natural, nitrate-free jerky
- Almond butter packets
- Shaker cup and protein powder (individual packets are great to have on hand)
- Freeze-dried/dehydrated veggies

Start a Food Log

Being accountable with your food is a great way to continue to engage your mind-set. There's no better way of doing this than with a food log. Here's why:

- **Your food log will clearly show you what you ate.** If you think you know exactly what you eat every day, you may be surprised at what sneaks in there. The pounds pile on because of the nibbles in between meals that you're not keeping track of. A soda here, a brownie there, the jumbo popcorn at the movie theater. You get the picture. Keeping track of everything you put in your body, no matter how small, will help you identify the extra you are putting in that might be adding the extra fat around your belly. Make sure you include all the little things, such as ghee, oil, and all the ingredients, in each dish.

EATING OUT WITHOUT BLOWING IT

Unprocessing your diet doesn't mean you can't eat out. That's just not practical (or fun). Healthier choices are always available no matter where you are. You can build a meal in a restaurant by choosing proteins, fats, and carbs using your hand as a measurement (see pages 69 to 74 for a refresher). I love fish, so I'll usually see what fish is on the menu. If I see it comes with pasta, I'll ask for extra vegetables instead. I know they've likely cooked their vegetables in fat, so I'm getting my fat in there. You could also build a meal on a salad by adding a protein, such as grilled chicken or fish. Ask for the dressing on the side and remember to tell them to leave out the cheese and croutons and, of course, the bread basket. If you are concerned about getting enough to eat, eat a little beforehand so you're sure to be satisfied by the end of the meal. If the portion looks huge, ask for half to be packed up before you take your first forkful. If you're visiting a friend or going to a party, offer to bring a dish to be sure you're covered. Don't be shy about sharing your goals with other people. Sharing helps keep you accountable, and most people will respect your goals.

- **Your food log will help you identify highs and lows in your day.** We all experience times of the day when our energy is lower, or where we might have brain fog, making it difficult to focus at work. Tracking what you eat enables you to connect what you put in your mouth and when with how you feel and lets you make changes accordingly. For example, if you know that every day around two p.m. you are craving sweets, or are exhausted, track it in your food log. Chances are, you'll find the culprit in what you're habitually eating.

- **Your food log will help you identify what you need to eat more of.** It's not just about what you're eating, it's also about what you're missing. For example, if you aren't up to speed with V3, that will be clear. If you are missing protein or fat in your meals, that will be clear, too. If you skip lunch or dinner, it may show up as oversnacking. Knowing what your deficit is can be just as useful as what you are eating too much of.

- **Your food log will keep you on track.** Writing down what you eat will make you want to make better choices and eat healthier foods. If you eat that slice of cake, you're going to have to write it down, and just that thought is a built-in braking system. Because it keeps you accountable, it will definitely make you think twice!

For many of us, committing to keeping a food log will be the missing link between our best intentions and reaching our weight-loss goals. And it's one of the easiest steps to skip over. "It feels tedious. . . . It interrupts the flow of my day. . . . It takes too much time. . . ." I've heard every excuse, but it's the people who don't do it who are the ones most likely to be disappointed with their results.

I've made a food log mandatory with every client I've worked with, and it's worked every time. But there was one client whom I just couldn't convince. She would tell me over and over again, "I'll send my food log to you tonight." But she never sent it. Whatever was holding her back was keeping her there; her stubbornness meant that those stubborn extra pounds weren't ready to come off. She hadn't made a decision. She was trying, but she wasn't ready to commit to the process. If this sounds familiar, revisit "Don't Just Try—Commit" (page 28). If one of your long-term goals is to feel great and start aging in reverse, make committing to a food log the daily goal that makes that long-term goal a reality. Don't forget to engage your mind-set!

Create your food log in a dedicated journal, on your phone or iPad (there are apps for that), or use the log on the following page (make several copies of it) to keep track of the food you put in your body. Choose whichever method is easiest for you. Use it for the full ten days, and if you find it useful, I invite you to use it daily going forward as you are working toward your fat-loss and health goals. Note: Don't cheat! No one needs to see your food log but you, and not keeping good track will only hurt you and get in the way of your goals.

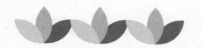

Food Log Date _____

Time	What I ate	How much?	How do I feel?

How much water did you drink? _____

Did you move your body today? _____

How do you feel about your food choices today? _____

Are there any changes you would make? _____

Did any particular meal make you feel particularly good or bad?

_____

Remember Your Decisions

Here's a quick refresher of my *Plan Your Plate* principles from pages 61 to 124:

☐ **Decision #1: I will make 100 percent unprocessed the base of my plate.**

No processed oils, sugar, artificial sweeteners, additives, preservatives, or convenience foods. *See page 61.*

☐ **Decision #2: I will balance my plate with protein, fats, and carbs.**

See pages 153 to 154 to for your list of choices and page 69 for the full rundown on proteins, fats, and carbs.

☐ **Decision #3: I will pack my plate with V3: value, volume, vegetables!**

Vegetables are your health insurance and your ticket to fast fat loss. Eat as many nonstarchy vegetables as you can! Enjoy a Daily Super Salad (page 227) and find creative ways to get more veggies in. *See page 75.*

☐ **Decision #4: I will keep my plate clear of added sugar (and its artificial imitators) and slow down on starchy carbs.**

Kick the sugar and fake stuff out of your life and limit your carbs. Fruit is the only sweetener for the next ten days, or until you've reached your fat-loss and overall health goals. *See page 79.*

❑ **Decision #5: I will clear my plate of inflammation triggers.**

Steer clear of dairy, grains, and legumes (including soy). *See page 86.*

❑ **Decision #6: I will perk up my plate with fermented foods.**

Add sauerkraut, pickles, cultured cashew cheese, and more to reap the life-giving benefits of ferments. *See page 93.*

❑ **Decision #7: I will hydrate my plate.**

Hydration comes not only from water but bone broth, veggies, and more veggies! *See page 99.*

❑ **Decision #8: I will fill my plate with anti-inflammatory superfoods.**

From sea vegetables to mushrooms and cacao, challenge yourself to add at least one superfood from the ten groups each day. *See page 104.*

❑ **Decision #9: I will supplement my plate.**

Add a select few supplements to reset your results. *See page 119.*

Build a Meal

The meal plan on pages 158 to 162 takes the guesswork out of what to put on your plate for the next ten days. Going unprocessed couldn't be more delicious! But I want you to think of these recipes as guidelines that you can change up based on your taste, preferences, and schedule. Using the following principles for building a meal, you can even skip the formal recipes altogether and come up with your own creations. Many of my clients have done so to accommodate their busy, often on-the-go lifestyles. There will be an abundance to choose from in your well-stocked unprocessed kitchen. Have fun and don't feel constrained!

Three Main Meals a Day

- Make one selection from the protein list.

- Make one selection from the fat list.

- Make one selection from the carb list.

- Fill your plate with as many of the unlimited carbs as you like.

Two Snacks or Treats a Day

- Select one serving from two of the three groups; for example, fruit and nuts (carb and fat) or sweet potato and chicken (carb and protein).

Count Carbs, Not Calories

- A small piece of fruit can be enjoyed with every meal, but starchy carbs (e.g., sweet potatoes and fresh corn) are limited to two meals a day. If you include a starchy carb in a meal, do not also include a fruit in that meal. You can have up to five pieces of fruit a day. See page 72 for further details.

- Eat fruits or starchy carbs with a fat or protein, never alone. Read about the blood sugar spikes eating carbs alone can cause on page 73.

- Note that strawberries, blueberries, raspberries, and blackberries are so low on the glycemic load that you can eat them unlimited the way you can eat vegetables.

- Eat as much as you like from the unlimited vegetable and berry list.

Proteins

Size of your palm, or 4 to 6 ounces

4 to 6 ounces fresh fish (e.g., salmon, halibut, sea bass, or tilapia)

4 to 6 ounces skinless chicken (breast or dark meat)

4 to 6 ounces skinless turkey (breast or dark meat)

4 to 6 ounces goose meat

4 ounces turkey bacon (nitrate-free)

4 ounces pork bacon (nitrate free; counts as your fat, too)

4 to 6 ounces turkey or chicken sausage

4 ounces beef, pork, or lamb (counts as your fat, too)

4 to 6 ounces goat

4 to 6 ounces venison, buffalo, boar, elk, or other game meat

1 (4- to 6-ounce) can tuna fish

½ cup (4 to 6 ounces) shellfish (e.g., shrimp, scallops, mussels, clams, crab, crayfish, lobster, octopus, or squid)

½ cup (4 to 6 ounces) sardines or herring

2 large eggs

6 large egg whites

Bone broth (page 163; this one's unlimited—sip away!)

Fats
Size of your thumb, or 1 to 2 tablespoons
(nuts are 6 to 10 pieces)

Avocado oil

Coconut butter

Coconut cream

Coconut oil

Extra-virgin olive oil

Ghee (page 168)

Olive oil or avocado
oil mayonnaise

Avocado

Almonds

Cashews

Hazelnuts

Macadamia nuts

Pecans

Pistachios

Walnuts

Flax seeds

Hemp seeds

Pumpkin seeds

Sesame seeds
(black and tan)

Sunflower seeds

Nut butters (*not*
peanut butter)

Seed butters

Starchy Carbs

Baked or roasted
potato (small)

Baked or roasted
sweet potato (small)

Corn on the cob
(small)

½ cup chopped
plantain

½ cup chopped
cassava (yuca)

Fruit
Size of your fist, or 1/2 cup (see *notes page 72*)

1 small apple

4 apricots

½ banana

½ cup cantaloupe

½ cup cherries

2 clementines

3 or 4 small fresh
figs

1 small grapefruit

½ cup grapes

1 cup honeydew
chunks

2 kiwis

½ mango

1 small orange

1 small peach

½ cup pineapple
chunks

2 plums

½ cup pomegranate
seeds

½ cup watermelon
chunks

Vegetables That You Can Eat Unlimited

Arugula

Asparagus

Basil

Beet greens

Beets

Bell peppers
(red, orange,
yellow, green)

Broccoli

Brussels sprouts

Cabbage

Carrots

Cauliflower

Celery

Chives

Cilantro

Collard greens

Cucumber

Dandelion greens

Eggplant

Endive

Fennel

Garlic

Ginger

Green beans

Iceberg lettuce

Kale

Mustard greens

Onions

Parsley

Radishes

Shallots

Snap peas

Snow peas

Spinach

Sprouts

Summer squash

Swiss chard

Tomatoes

Turnips

Watercress

Zucchini

Berries That You Can Eat Unlimited

Blackberries

Blueberries

Raspberries

Strawberries

Free Foods

Bone Broth (page 163)

Crunchy Dulse Chips
(page 231)

Dill pickles (page 231)

Green Salsa (page
173) or another
unprocessed salsa

Sauerkraut (page 174)

Unlimited Add-ons

Lemon

Lime

Salsa

Vinegar (any, except
malt vinegar)

Mustard (check that
it's gluten-free)

Dried herbs and spices

Fresh spices

Raw cacao powder

Beverages

Flat water	Unsweetened iced or	Bone Broth (page 163)
Sparkling water	hot tea	
Super Water (page	Coffee	
165)		

Notes About the Recipes

Make the most of the recipes by keeping in mind the following:

- Recipes typically serve two, but if it's just you, you can save the rest for a second meal or freeze it. And most recipes can double easily if you're feeding a family (family members who are not looking to lose weight may add a serving of grains or legumes to increase the calories). Smoothies serve one because smoothies are best made fresh. Doubling them is a cinch if you've got someone to share with.

- I have not used beef, pork, or lamb in my recipes because I personally do not eat these meats. That doesn't mean that they aren't healthy options, though! Feel free to swap in another meat (preferably grass-fed and organic) for the poultry, fish, or shrimp. Beef, pork, and lamb count as both a protein and a fat.

- Nutritional values include optional ingredients but not swaps. All swaps are well within the guidelines of the plan.

- A protein serving is 4 to 6 ounces; most recipes use the higher number to ensure that you're full. If you feel that will be too much, scale the number down.

- Enjoy your Super Salad (page 227) every day, but it doesn't matter what time of day. You could even have it with breakfast or as a between-meal snack.

- Feel free to swap lunch with dinner or mix and match from different days of the week.

- If you're missing bread, crumble up an Everything Cracker (page 229) or other grain-free cracker to sprinkle over a soup or salad.

- For a carb-light wrap, use a sheet of nori, a collard leaf, or a coconut wrap (a wrap made entirely of coconut; it counts as a fat).

- Include Cauliflower Rice (page 176) as a very low-carb grain alternative with any recipe (remember, nonstarchy vegetables are unlimited!).

- Squeeze a big batch of lemons and limes and chop multiple garlic cloves in the beginning of the week. You'll thank yourself for the prep time it saves you.

- Poach chicken and shrimp and bake a few sweet potatoes in advance to have them ready for your recipes. You'll save tons of time getting your meals together.

- Cook with love and you'll taste the difference!

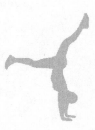

10-Day Meal Plan

Note: Snacks, treats, Super Salad, and Bone Broth can be enjoyed any time of day. When you're feeling hungry would be the best time!

DAY 1	DAY 2
Breakfast Stovetop Sweet Potato Hash and Eggs (page 182)	**Breakfast** Turkey Bacon and Egg Breakfast Muffin (page 183)
Lunch Pesto Turkey Burgers (page 207) 1 serving of fruit	**Lunch** Lemony Kale and Chicken Salad (page 196)
Snack 2 Everything Crackers (page 229) or other grain-free crackers with 1 tablespoon Creamy Cashew Cheese (page 170) *or* 1 fruit and 6 to 8 nuts	**Snack** Nori Grabber (page 243) *or* Cheesy Date (page 244)
Daily Super Salad (page 227; any time of day)	**Daily Super Salad** (page 227; any time of day)
Sip on unlimited Bone Broth (page 163)	**Sip on unlimited Bone Broth** (page 163)
Dinner Hot and Sour Egg Drop Soup (page 222) Chicken and Spinach Loaded Sweet Potatoes (page 209)	**Dinner** Hot and Sour Egg Drop Soup (page 222) Seared Scallops and Turmeric Cauliflower Rice (page 214)
Treat Almond Protein Bite (page 237)	**Treat** Almond Protein Bite (page 237)

DAY 3

Breakfast
Turkey Sausage with Two-Minute
Wilted Greens (page 184)
1 serving of fruit

Lunch
Thai-Style Shrimp, Cucumber,
and Pineapple Salad (page 199)

Snack
Coconut Chip Trail Mix
(page 238)

Daily Super Salad
(page 227; any time of day)

Sip on unlimited Bone Broth
(page 163)

Dinner
Ginger Chicken Soup (page 226)
Baked Whitefish with Green Salsa
and Fresh Corn (page 216)

Treat
Banana Nut Muffin (page 239)

DAY 4

Breakfast
Sesame Asparagus with Fried Eggs
(page 187)
1 serving of fruit

Lunch
Scallion Chicken Salad with No-
Peanut Peanut Sauce (page 197)

Snack
Coconut Chip Trail Mix
(page 238)

Daily Super Salad
(page 227; any time of day)

Sip on unlimited Bone Broth
(page 163)

Dinner
Ginger Chicken Soup (page 226)
Zucchini Noodles and Shrimp
with Loaded Greens Pesto
(page 217)

Treat
Banana Nut Muffin (page 239)

DAY 5

Breakfast
Very Berry Smoothie Bowl
    (page 190)

Lunch
Spicy Sausage, Pepper, and Onion
    Bowl (page 206)

Snack
2 Everything Crackers (page 229)
    or other grain-free cracker with
    1 tablespoon Creamy Cashew
    Cheese (page 170)

or

1 fruit and 6 to 8 nuts

Daily Super Salad
(page 227; any time of day)

Sip on unlimited Bone Broth
(page 163)

Dinner
Soothing Butternut Squash Soup
    (page 223)
Garlicky Shrimp, Shiitake, and
    Broccoli Stir-fry (page 218)

Treat
1 piece Raw Cacao Fudge
    (page 240)

DAY 6

Breakfast
Carrot Cake Colada Smoothie
    (page 192)

Lunch
Simplest Taco Salad Bowl
    (page 207)

Snack
Nori Grabber (page 243)

or

Celery sticks with 1 tablespoon nut
    butter

Daily Super Salad
(page 227; any time of day)

Sip on unlimited Bone Broth
(page 163)

Dinner
Soothing Butternut Squash Soup
    (page 223)
Broiled Salmon with Blackened
    Scallions and Loaded Greens
    Pesto (page 220)

Treat
1 piece Raw Cacao Fudge
    (page 240)

DAY 7

Breakfast
Dilly Smoked Salmon Scramble
(page 186)
1 serving of fruit

Lunch
Sea Vegetable Shrimp Lettuce
Wraps (page 203)

Snack
Zucchini and Roasted Yellow
Pepper Hummus (page 233)
with 2 Everything Crackers
(page 229) or other grain-free
crackers

Daily Super Salad
(page 227; any time of day)

Sip on unlimited Bone Broth
(page 163)

Dinner
Tomato, Zucchini, and Basil Soup
(page 224)
Oven-Baked Hot Wings and Sweet
Potatoes (page 210)

Treat
1 Frozen Fig and Cocoa
Cheesecake Bite (page 241)

DAY 8

Breakfast
Herb, Shiitake, and Spinach
Omelet (page 189)
1 serving of fruit

Lunch
Citrus Tuna Poke Bowl (page 204)

Snack
Zucchini and Roasted Yellow
Pepper Hummus (page 233)
with 2 Everything Crackers
(page 229) or other grain-free
crackers

Daily Super Salad
(page 227; any time of day)

Sip on unlimited Bone Broth
(page 163)

Dinner
Tomato, Zucchini, and Basil Soup
(page 224)
Turkey Tacos (page 212)

Treat
1 Frozen Fig and Cocoa
Cheesecake Bite (page 241)

DAY 9

Breakfast
Super Green Smoothie (page 193)

Lunch
Tahini Tuna Salad (page 201)

Snack
Mushroom Jerky (page 236)

Daily Super Salad
(page 227; any time of day)

Sip on unlimited Bone Broth
(page 163)

Dinner
Neglected Veggie Stem Soup
    (page 225)
Smoky Chocolate Turkey Chili
    (page 213)

Treat
Strawberries and Coconut
    Whipped Cream (page 242)

DAY 10

Breakfast
Cinnamon Chocolate Smoothie
    (page 195)

Lunch
Mango, Avocado, and Arugula
    Shrimp Salad (page 200)

Snack
Mushroom Jerky (page 236)

Daily Super Salad
(page 227; any time of day)

Sip on unlimited Bone Broth
(page 163)

Dinner
Neglected Veggie Stem Soup
    (page 225)
One-Pan Chicken Fajitas
    (page 211)

Treat
Strawberries and Coconut
    Whipped Cream (page 242)

The Recipes

Essentials

Bone Broth

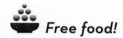 *Free food!*

ONE SIP OF this savory elixir and your body will tell you it is exactly what it needs. Cooking with bone broth is one of the easiest and most enjoyable ways of getting solid nutrition into your body on a daily basis. Bone broth is a fantastic source of protein, collagen, hydration, and vitamins and minerals, and it improves digestion, boosts immunity, curbs appetite, and even makes your hair and nails look better! Read more about this superfood on page 115.

Making a commitment to making bone broth is a great reason to go out and get a slow cooker if you don't already have one (you can also make bone broth in an Instant Pot). This recipe involves only a few minutes of hands-on prep, but if time or space is a concern, there are many good-quality brands of bone broth on the market to choose from.

MAKES 4 QUARTS

3 pounds organic chicken, beef, pork, or lamb bones
1 large onion, roughly chopped
1 large carrot, roughly chopped
1 celery rib, including leaves, roughly chopped
3 garlic cloves
1 sheet kombu (see page 108; optional)

(Continues)

(Bone Broth Continued)

1 tablespoon cider vinegar
    1 tablespoon black peppercorns
    1 teaspoon ground turmeric
    2 teaspoons sea salt, plus more to taste

Place the bones in a slow cooker. Add 4 quarts of water and the remaining ingredients, cover, and cook on LOW for 12 to 24 hours. Alternatively, place the bones in a large stockpot. Add 4 quarts of water and bring to a boil. Boil for 5 minutes, skimming off any foam that rises to the top. Add the remaining ingredients, bring to a simmer, then lower the heat to very low, cover, and cook at a bare simmer for 12 hours, topping up with water if the level falls below the top of the bones.

Remove the bones with tongs, then strain the broth through a fine-mesh strainer lined with cheesecloth into a heatproof bowl. Use immediately, or allow to cool and pour into containers. It will keep for up to 1 week in the refrigerator or in the freezer for up to 6 months.

> **Each serving (1½ cups):**
> 15 g protein, 0 g fat, 1 g carbs, 71 calories

• Neglected Veggie Alert!
Save kitchen scraps, including parsley and cilantro stems; carrot, celery, and zucchini ends; and shiitake mushroom stems to add more flavor and nutrition to your broth.

Become a Better Cook in an Instant

Bone broth makes any recipe you use it in taste better. You will instantly become a better cook just by using it in your cooking!

Super Water

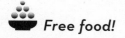 *Free food!*

SKIP THOSE ENHANCED colored waters you find at the supermarket. They will only empty your pocketbook and fill your belly with more sugar than the vitamins they claim to contain. You can make your own version at home with just two ingredients: fruit and water. What a sweet way to keep on track with your daily hydration!

Chances are, you've already got the makings of Super Water at home in your fridge—just about any fruits, herbs, and spices will work, and cucumber will add a cool, refreshing note. If you're exercising hard, try adding a pinch of salt to your Super Water to replace lost electrolytes. Note that there's no nutritional data for this recipe, since it will vary based on the fruits and herbs you choose, but know that you can drink it freely!

MAKES 2 QUARTS

About 2 cups chopped or sliced fruit
Handful of herbs, such as mint, lemon balm, rosemary,
    or lavender

Put the fruit in the bottom of a 2-quart jar. Lightly smash it with a wooden spoon to start to release some of the juice. Gently bruise the herbs by rolling them between your hands, then add them to the jar. Top with water, place in the refrigerator, and leave to infuse for at least 4 hours or overnight. Serve over ice. Top up with water as you empty the jar; the mixture will keep for up to 4 days.

Super Water Combo Ideas

| Pineapple and Sage | Mixed Berry and Lime | Grapefruit and Thyme |
| Orange and Strawberry | Cucumber, Lemon, and Mint | Apple, Cranberry, and Cinnamon |

Flavored Ice Cubes

Jazz up your ice and add spunk to your water! Who knew hydration could be so beautiful? Here are some ideas:

Floral freezers: Set unsprayed edible flowers, such as violets, in an ice cube tray, top with water, and freeze.

Herby ice: Fill an ice cube tray with herb leaves, such as mint or basil, top with water, and freeze.

Pure fruit ice: Freeze whole chunks of pineapple or grapes.

Berry coolers: Fill an ice cube tray with berries, add water, and freeze.

Citrus chillers: Freeze lemon or lime slices.

Must-have melon: Freeze melon balls.

Caffeinated cubes: Freeze brewed coffee or tea.

Coco cubes: Freeze coconut water.

Maple cubes: Freeze maple water (see sidebar, page 194).

Super Water cubes: Freeze Super Water (page 165) into cubes.

Almond Milk

WHILE CARTONS OF packaged almond milk are convenient, once you try homemade, you just might be hooked on its fresh, pure flavor. It's easy to make; you'll just need to plan in advance, as the recipe calls for soaking almonds in water for at least twelve hours. It's best if you have a high-speed blender, but you can also make this in a regular blender.

MAKES ABOUT 1 QUART

1½ cups almonds

Place the almonds in a medium-size bowl and add water to cover by a couple of inches. Cover with a kitchen towel and soak for at least 12 hours or up to 24 hours. Drain the almonds, then place them in a blender, add 4 cups of fresh water, and blend until smooth, about 2 minutes. Strain through a nut milk bag or strainer lined with cheesecloth into a bowl; squeeze on the pulp to extract all the liquid. The almond milk will keep refrigerated for up to 4 days.

Each serving (½ cup):
1 g protein, 1 g fat, 1 g carbs, 17 calories

- *Swap Outs*
  Use another nut, such as cashews or Brazil nuts, and add flavorings, such as pure vanilla extract or ground cinnamon or cardamom, to change things up.

- *Supercharge It!*
  Save the almond pulp that remains after straining your almond milk and add to your smoothies for extra fiber.

Ghee

COOK BUTTER TO brown the milk solids that separate out and you're left with pure golden butterfat. That's ghee, a form of clarified butter and a fat the color of sunshine. While ghee is technically a dairy product, it can be included in most dairy-free diets (except for people who are extremely sensitive to the casein and lactose in dairy). Ghee has a higher smoke point than olive oil, making it a good choice for high-heat cooking.

Ghee is rich in fat-soluble (meaning you need fat to absorb them) vitamins A, E, and K. It also contains butyrate, a short-chain fatty acid that supports digestive health, and conjugated linoleic acid, another fatty acid that fights off inflammation and may even help with fat loss. The fats in ghee help feed your brain, so choosing this superfat over processed oils, such as canola and vegetable oil, is a no-brainer!

MAKES ABOUT 2 CUPS

1 pound unsalted butter, cubed

Line a strainer with several layers of cheesecloth or a nut milk bag and set aside.

Heat the butter in a medium-size saucepan over medium heat until melted. Reduce the heat to very low and cook without stirring for about 30 minutes. As the butter turns to ghee, the water will evaporate, the butter will foam, and you'll hear tiny crackling noises. The ghee is ready when the foam is almost gone, the crackling turns into a boiling sound, and the butterfat is a pure golden color with the milk solids browned and settled at the bottom.

Remove the saucepan from the heat and let the ghee cool without stirring until just warm. Pour through the lined strainer and discard the solids (this is the dairy part of the butter). Pour the ghee into a glass jar and allow to cool completely. It will keep, covered, at room temperature for up to 1 month or in the refrigerator for up to 4 months.

Each serving (1 tablespoon):
0 g protein, 15 g fat, 0 g carbs, 135 calories

Basic Nut Butter

MAKING NUT BUTTER is fun and easy, and you get to decide which nuts to use (my favorite is a combo of macadamia and cashew) and whether you want yours chunky or smooth. If you want to make chunky nut butter, reserve a handful of nuts, add them at the end, and pulse a few times to desired chunkiness. If you prefer a raw nut butter, or to save time, skip the roasting step.

MAKES ABOUT 2½ CUPS

4 cups raw almonds, cashews, macadamia nuts, or other nuts
½ teaspoon sea salt, or to taste
1 tablespoon extra-virgin olive oil, plus more if needed

Preheat the oven to 350°F.

Spread the nuts over a baking sheet and roast for 7 to 10 minutes, stirring once halfway through, until the nuts are lightly browned. Remove from the oven, transfer to a food processor, and allow to cool.

Once the nuts have cooled, process them for about 2 minutes, stopping to scrape down the sides of the processor a couple of times, until the nuts are crumbly. Add the salt and oil and process for 5 to 7 minutes, to your desired smoothness, stopping to scrape the sides a few times. As the nuts turn to nut butter, the whole thing will gather into a ball, and as the oils continue to release, the ball will loosen into a fairly smooth puree. Note that this can take some time, so just be patient—it will work! Transfer the nut butter to a lidded jar. It will keep in the refrigerator for up to 4 months.

Each serving of almond butter (1 tablespoon):
3 g protein, 7 g fat, 3 g carbs, 86 calories

Creamy Cashew Cheese

WHEN CASHEWS ARE soaked in water and then blended, they add a supercreamy base to hummus (page 233), cheesecake (page 241), and this tangy, dairy-free cream cheese. This cheese goes through fermentation, which here simply means adding probiotic powder and leaving it on the counter for a couple days. Feel free to add herbs and spices to vary the flavor and up the superfood content. Make sure to purchase a probiotic powder labeled *dairy-free* to keep your cheese dairy-free. If you don't find a powdered probiotic, simply empty a few probiotic capsules.

MAKES 1 CUP

1½ cups raw cashews
1 teaspoon probiotic powder
½ teaspoon sea salt

Place the cashews in a medium-size bowl and add water to cover. Cover with a dish towel and soak for at least 4 hours or up to 12 hours. Drain.

In a small high-speed blender or food processor, combine the cashews, ¼ cup of water, the probiotic powder, and salt and blend until silky smooth, 3 to 5 minutes, stopping to scrape the sides of the machine as needed and adding more water if it's too thick. Place in a jar or container, loosely cover, and leave on the counter to ferment for 2 to 3 days, stirring once or twice a day to prevent a skin from forming on top. The cheese is done when it's as tangy as you like it. It will keep in the refrigerator for up to 2 weeks.

Each serving (2 tablespoons):
4 g protein, 11 g fat, 6 g carbs, 136 calories

TIP: You'll get the silkiest results by using a blender; add more time if using a food processor.

Essential Salad Dressing

THIS DRESSING TAKES under five minutes to make, and it's tastier, healthier, and more economical than the bottled kind from the store, which is usually filled with sugar and stabilizers. It's perfect for all your salad dressing needs, in particular your Daily Super Salad (page 227). Double or triple the batch and keep it on hand!

MAKES ½ CUP

¼ cup extra-virgin olive oil
1 tablespoon cider vinegar
1 tablespoon white wine vinegar
1 teaspoon Dijon mustard
1 garlic clove, pressed through a garlic press
1 tablespoon freshly squeezed lemon juice, or to taste
¼ teaspoon sea salt, or to taste
¼ teaspoon freshly ground black pepper, or to taste

In a jar with a lid, combine all the ingredients and shake until emulsified. Taste and adjust the seasonings if needed. The dressing will keep, refrigerated, for up to 1 week.

Each serving (2 tablespoons):
0 g protein, 14 g fat, 1 g carbs, 125 calories

Swap Outs
- Add fresh or dried herbs, such as parsley, cilantro, tarragon, or rosemary.
- Swap out the white wine vinegar for red.

Supercharge It!
Add ½ teaspoon of dulse granules to the dressing.

Loaded Greens Pesto

PESTO IS ONE of my top freezer staples because it's so versatile: pull some out and serve over fish (page 220), zucchini noodles (page 217), or scrambled eggs and you've made yourself a meal. This pesto skips the Parm to go dairy-free (trust me, you won't miss it), and basil shares the stage with two potent detoxifiers, parsley and cilantro.

MAKES 1½ CUPS

3 garlic cloves, peeled
1 cup walnut halves
¾ teaspoon sea salt, or to taste
¼ teaspoon freshly ground black pepper, or to taste
2 tablespoons freshly squeezed lemon juice, or to taste
2 cups fresh basil leaves
1 cup chopped fresh flat-leaf parsley leaves
1 cup chopped fresh cilantro
⅔ cup extra-virgin olive oil

In a food processor with the motor running, drop the garlic through the hole in the top to mince. Add the walnuts, salt, and pepper and process until coarsely ground. Add the lemon juice, basil, parsley, and cilantro and process to mince the herbs. With the motor still running, drizzle in the oil through the hole in the top to incorporate. If the mixture is too thick, add a little water. Transfer to a container, cover, and store in the refrigerator for up to 1 week or in the freezer for up to 3 months.

Each serving (2 tablespoons):
2 g protein, 18 g fat, 2 g carbs, 167 calories

● *Neglected Veggie Alert!*
Include both the leaves and stems from the parsley and cilantro and toss the basil stems into Super Water (page 165).

- *Swap Outs*
  - Use other greens, such as arugula or mint.
  - Swap in pecans or pumpkin seeds for the walnuts.

> ### Freeze Pesto for Future Meals
>
> To freeze pesto, line a baking sheet with parchment or waxed paper and spoon 2-tablespoon heaps of the pesto onto the sheet. Freeze until solid, about 2 hours, then pop into a freezer bag for storage. Or freeze in ice cube trays.

Green Salsa

 Free food!

THIS IS THE condiment you'll find in Mexican restaurants alongside chips that tempt you to dip. For your unprocessed diet, it's equally at home over fish, stirred into scrambled eggs, or as a quick sauce for shredded chicken (see page 207). Tart tomatillos look like small green tomatoes with a papery husk that you remove before using them. You'll find them in the produce aisle of your grocery store or a store that sells Mexican ingredients. Bonus: Because this salsa is so low in calories, it's a free food that you can pour liberally over your food or use as a dip for vegetable sticks.

MAKES ABOUT 2 CUPS

1 pound tomatillos, husked and rinsed well
½ small red onion, coarsely chopped
2 garlic cloves, peeled
1 jalapeño chile, stemmed and cut in half (seeded if you like)
1 teaspoon sea salt, or to taste
½ cup chopped fresh cilantro leaves and stems

(Continues)

(Green Salsa Continued)

Combine the tomatillos and red onion in a small saucepan and add water to cover. Place over high heat and bring to a boil. Lower the heat to medium and simmer for about 5 minutes, until the tomatillos begin to dull in color.

Using a slotted spoon, transfer the tomatillos and red onion to a blender or food processor, reserving the cooking liquid in the pan. Add the garlic, jalapeño, and salt and pulse until smooth and pourable. Add the cilantro and pulse to incorporate it. Add some of the reserved cooking liquid if the salsa is too thick. Serve immediately, or transfer to a container, cover, and store in the refrigerator, where it will keep for up to 1 week.

> **Each serving (½ cup):**
> **1 g protein, 1 g fat, 8 g carbs, 44 calories**

Sauerkraut

AFTER READING ABOUT the amazing benefits of probiotic-rich fermented foods, from better digestion to reduced cravings and fat loss (see pages 93 to 98), you probably are excited to try your hand at making your own!* Sauerkraut is an easy introduction to fermentation (my Creamy Cashew Cheese on page 170 is another), and you might consider inviting friends and family in on the fun—have everyone bring a head of cabbage and a 1-quart jar and everybody will go home with the makings of sauerkraut. Sauerkraut has amazing staying power—about a year—so feel free to double the recipe to keep your fridge filled with live and active cultures.

MAKES 2 QUARTS

---

* If life gets in the way, know that there are many great options at your natural food store—look for the words *live, raw,* or *contains living cultures* on the label.

1 medium-size head cabbage (about 2½ pounds)
1 tablespoon fine sea salt
1½ teaspoons caraway seeds (optional)

Remove the outer leaves from the cabbage and set them aside. Cut the cabbage in half and remove the core and root end from each half; set those aside. Quarter the cabbage, slice it into thin lengthwise strips, then chop the strips. Place the cabbage and salt in a large nonreactive bowl (stainless steel is okay). Using your hands, mix, squeeze, and massage the salt into the cabbage for about 5 minutes to release water from it and start to create a salty brine. Set the cabbage aside for 20 to 30 minutes (or up to 4 hours) to allow the salt to draw out the liquid and further soften the cabbage. Stir in the caraway seeds, if using.

Pack the cabbage into a 2-quart glass jar a little at a time, leaving at least 1 inch of space remaining at the top; after each addition, press it down with your hand to release more water. You'll know you've released enough water when the cabbage is submerged in its brine. Place the cabbage core on top of the cabbage. Roll up the reserved outer cabbage leaves and stuff them on top of the cabbage core. This will keep the sauerkraut under the brine. Loosely cover with the lid, place the jar on a rimmed plate to catch any potential overflow, and set aside in a cool place out of direct sunlight to ferment. Check every day to make sure the cabbage is covered with brine, pressing down on it or adding a little extra brine if it isn't. Your sauerkraut will be ready in 1 to 4 weeks, depending on how warm it is in your kitchen and how tangy you like your sauerkraut. Cover and store in the refrigerator, where it will keep for about 1 year.

Each serving (¼ cup): 0 g protein, 0 g fat, 2 g carbs, 11 calories

- ● *Neglected Veggie Alert!*
  Save the outer leaves and cores from your cabbage and use them as a final layer for the kraut jar.

- ● *Add V3*
  Include shredded beets or carrots or add fresh herbs, such as cilantro, dill, or mint.

Go for the Good Bacteria

Check your cabbage every day as it ferments. The key to keeping out harmful bacteria is to always keep the cabbage covered in brine, so if it isn't, simply press down on it to submerge it. If any mold develops, don't freak out and throw it out. Simply remove the part of the cabbage that came into contact with the mold. Rest assured that your kraut jar is an anaerobic environment where it's almost impossible for harmful bacteria to take root.

Cauliflower Rice

RICE-SIZE BITS OF cauliflower are a trusty grain-free cook's companion. Cauliflower, like rice, is a culinary blank slate and takes on the flavors of any food it's paired with. Serve your cauliflower rice raw in a salad or as a side, or cooked in place of your standard bowl of rice. Make sure not to overdo it in the food processor, or your cauliflower will turn to a puree.

MAKES ABOUT 6 CUPS

1 large head cauliflower (about 2 pounds)
1 tablespoon extra-virgin olive oil or ghee (if cooking the rice)
1 teaspoon sea salt (if cooking the rice)

Trim the inner core from each cauliflower quarter and cut it into 1-inch florets. Cut the core into 1-inch pieces.

Add half of the cauliflower to a food processor and process until broken down into pieces the size of rice, about ⅛ inch, scraping down the sides as needed. Transfer to a bowl. Remove any large pieces of cauliflower and add them back to the processor. Repeat with the remaining cauliflower and add it to the bowl.

If you're serving your cauliflower rice raw, it's ready. To cook it, heat the oil in a large skillet over medium heat. Add the cauliflower and salt, cover, and cook for about 5 minutes, until crisp-tender. Serve immediately, or allow to cool, cover, and refrigerate for up to 1 week.

Each serving (raw; 1½ cups):
4 g protein, 1 g fat, 11 g carbs, 57 calories
. . .
Each serving (cooked; 1½ cups):
4 g protein, 4 g fat, 11 g carbs, 87 calories

TIP: *Purchase packaged cauliflower rice for convenience. You'll find it in the produce aisle. Cauliflower rice freezes well; pack up single-serving bags and have them ready for meal making.*

Move Over, Kale— There's a New Superveg in Town

Over the past few years, kale has become a superstar superfood. But did you know that cauliflower is in the same family as kale? They are known as crucifers, and they are powerful anticancer foods. While kale can transform into chips, cauliflower can also do neat tricks, such as change its shape to rice and even pizza. Cauliflower rice is a perfect sub for "real" rice for those of us watching our carbs, and its short list of nutrients is impressive, including folate, thiamine, riboflavin, niacin, magnesium, potassium, and vitamin B_6. Cauliflower is also great roasted: cut a head into florets, toss with extra-virgin olive oil, salt, and pepper, spread out over a baking sheet, and bake in a preheated 450°F oven for about 30 minutes, until softened and well browned.

Poached Chicken

POACH YOUR POULTRY in advance and you'll have juicy, tender chicken ready for soups, salads, and mains all week long. Or shred it and freeze it in preportioned bags. To flavor your poaching liquid, add garlic cloves, a bay leaf, and/or black peppercorns. You can make any amount of chicken following this method.

MAKES 2 POUNDS

2 pounds boneless or bone-in chicken breasts or legs
1 teaspoon sea salt

Place the chicken in a large saucepan. Add the salt and cold water to cover by about 1 inch. Place over medium-high heat and bring to a boil, skimming off any foam that rises to the top. Lower the heat to low, cover, and cook for to 15 to 20 minutes, until the chicken is cooked through and registers 165°F on an instant-read thermometer. Remove the chicken from the pan and place it on a cutting board. Use as directed in your recipes. It will keep, covered, in the refrigerator for up to 5 days or in the freezer for up to 2 months.

Each serving (6 ounces):
38 g protein, 4 g fat, 0 g carbs, 198 calories

TIP: Reheat poached chicken in Bone Broth (page 163) to add flavor to both the chicken and broth.

● *Neglected Veggie Alert!*
Add leftover herb stems to flavor the poaching liquid.

Poached Shrimp

SHRIMP IS A superfast protein option, and when you poach a batch of shrimp, you'll be one step closer to filling your lunch box and one step farther away from ordering in. Feel free to add lemon or lime slices, black peppercorns, or herb stems, to flavor the poaching liquid. Scale the amount of shrimp up or down as needed.

MAKES 12 OUNCES

12 ounces uncooked peeled shrimp
½ teaspoon sea salt

Bring a large pot of water to a boil. Add the shrimp, stir, remove from the heat, and cover. Leave for 10 minutes, then drain, pat dry with paper towels, and use as directed in your recipes. It will keep covered in the refrigerator for up to 4 days.

Each serving (6 ounces):
29 g protein, 2 g fat, 2 g carbs, 154 calories

Selecting Shrimp

Shrimp is a fast and easy source of protein, and it contains vitamin D, selenium for heart protection, and energy-boosting B vitamins. When time is tight, precooked shrimp plus salad makes a meal in less time it would take to get through the drive-through! To make sure your shrimp is as healthy as possible, choose wild whenever possible. Most shrimp we eat is from industrial shrimp farms from faraway waters and are processed with pesticides and other chemicals, not a plus for an unprocessed foods diet. Wild shrimp is not always available, so when you find it in your grocery store, pick up extra to stock your freezer.

Sweet Potatoes,
Baked or Steamed

SWEET POTATOES ARE my starchy carb of choice, as their orange color indicates the powerful carotenoid beta-carotene, which protects us from free radical damage, supports our immune system, and lowers our risk of heart disease and cancer. And although they are a carb, their high fiber content helps regulate blood sugar and keeps you full to support your fat-loss efforts. That's why I like to bake or steam a few in the beginning of the week and reheat them as an easy add to breakfast, lunch, or dinner. Cooked sweet potatoes will last for up to 4 days stored in the fridge.

> **As many sweet potatoes as you like**
> **Extra-virgin olive oil (about ½ teaspoon per potato); if steaming, no oil is needed**

To bake sweet potatoes: Preheat the oven to 400°F and line a baking sheet with aluminum foil.

Scrub the sweet potatoes and pat them dry with a dish towel. Prick them with a fork in three or four places. Rub the sweet potatoes with oil, then arrange them on the prepared baking sheet with at least 2 inches of space apart.

Bake until a knife tip slips easily into the center of a sweet potato and goes all the way through, between 30 minutes and 1 hour depending on the size of your sweet potatoes. Serve as directed in your recipes.

To steam sweet potatoes: Peel the sweet potatoes and cut them into roughly 1-inch chunks. Place them in a steamer basket set over a pot filled with a couple inches of simmering water. Cover and steam until tender when poked with knife or fork, 15 to 20 minutes. Remove from the steamer and serve as directed in your recipes.

1 medium-size (4-ounce) sweet potato:
2 g protein, 0 g fat, 24 g carbs, 103 calories

Coconut Whipped Cream

COCONUT WHIPPED CREAM delivers dairy-free satisfaction while feeding your body the good fats that it needs. This recipe requires an electric hand mixer, and you'll need to plan an hour ahead to chill the coconut cream, mixing bowl, and beaters before beating the coconut into cream. Enjoy a spoonful over coffee, or with berries or another fruit for a satisfying treat. You'll never go back to the processed stuff from the can!

MAKES 1 HEAPING CUP

1 cup coconut cream (see Note)
¼ teaspoon pure vanilla extract (optional)
Pinch of sea salt (optional)

Put the coconut cream into a large bowl and add the vanilla and salt, if using. Put the bowl in the refrigerator; put the beaters from a hand mixer in the refrigerator, too. Leave them there to chill for 1 to 2 hours, then whip for about 3 minutes, until creamy and smooth. Leftover coconut whipped cream will keep for up to 1 week, covered, in the refrigerator. If it solidifies, simply rewhip it to make it light and fluffy again.

**Each serving (2 heaping tablespoons):
0 g protein, 6 g fat, 1 g carbs, 60 calories**

Note: Use unsweetened coconut cream from the can or one can of full-fat coconut milk (lite varieties won't work). If using coconut milk, spoon the coconut cream from the top of the can, leaving any clear liquid at the bottom. Most coconut cream recipes call for refrigerating the can and then scooping out the cream, but I find that it gets so solid that it becomes hard to scoop out and measure. Reserve the liquid for use in other recipes or add to smoothies or breakfast bowls.

Breakfast

Stovetop Sweet Potato Hash and Eggs

FILLED WITH SUPERFOODS from mushrooms to turmeric, this hearty hash is topped off with eggs for a one-dish meal. Serve it straight from the pan for an eye-popping presentation.

SERVES 2

2 tablespoons extra-virgin olive oil, coconut oil, or ghee
1 small red onion, chopped
½ green bell pepper, chopped
4 shiitake mushrooms, stemmed and chopped
2 garlic cloves, minced
½ teaspoon ground cumin
¼ teaspoon ground turmeric
¼ teaspoon freshly ground black pepper
1 cup cubed sweet potato (¼-inch cubes)
¼ teaspoon plus a large pinch of sea salt
4 large eggs
2 cups arugula leaves

Heat the oil in a large skillet with a lid over medium heat. Add the onion and green pepper and cook until starting to soften, about 5 minutes. Add the mushrooms and cook for another 2 minutes, or until softened. Add the garlic and cook for 1 minute.

Add the cumin, turmeric, and black pepper and cook for 1 minute to bring out their flavors. Stir in the sweet potato and ¼ teaspoon of the salt and stir to coat the sweet potato in the spices. Cook until the sweet potato is softened and starting to brown, about 8 minutes. If the pan starts looking dry, add 1 to 2 tablespoons of water and cover the pan to finish cooking.

Make four wells in the sweet potatoes, crack the eggs into the wells, and sprinkle with the remaining pinch of salt. Cover and cook until the whites are set and the yolks are cooked to your liking. Serve straight from the skillet with the arugula on the side.

Each serving: 16 g protein, 24 g fat, 24 g carbs, 368 calories

● *Neglected Veggie Alert!*
Save your shiitake mushroom stems and add them to a pot of simmering bone broth.

Turkey Bacon and Egg Breakfast Muffins

BACON MAKES AN irresistible "cup" for your eggs, satisfying the urge for muffins while keeping your breakfast grain-free. The recipe doubles easily; wrap the muffins individually in foil and reheat in the toaster oven.

SERVES 2

Extra-virgin olive oil or coconut oil cooking spray
6 slices turkey bacon
4 large eggs
½ teaspoon sea salt
¼ teaspoon ground turmeric
¼ teaspoon freshly ground black pepper
6 cherry tomatoes, quartered (or cut into eighths if large)
2 scallions, white and green parts, finely chopped
4 tablespoons Creamy Cashew Cheese (page 170)

Preheat the oven to 375°F. Coat six wells of a muffin pan with cooking spray.

(Continues)

(*Turkey Bacon and Egg Breakfast Muffins* Continued)

Line each muffin cup with a slice of bacon, covering the sides and bottom.

In a medium-size bowl, beat the eggs, then beat in the salt, turmeric, and pepper. Put the cherry tomatoes and scallions in the bottom of the muffin cups, then pour the beaten egg into the cups. Bake for about 30 minutes, until the eggs are set and the bacon is cooked through. Top with the cheese and serve.

Each serving: 23 g protein, 25 g fat, 10 g carbs, 370 calories

● *Swaps Outs*
- Swap pork bacon for the turkey bacon. Omit the Creamy Cashew Cheese, as pork bacon counts as both a protein and a fat.
- If you don't have Creamy Cashew Cheese, top the muffins with ½ mashed avocado.
- Add minced onion or bell pepper in place of the scallions.

● *Supercharge It!*
Make use of your second oven rack to add V3 to your meal. While the muffins are baking, tear the leaves of ½ bunch of kale and toss with a small amount of extra-virgin olive oil and a pinch of sea salt. Spread out over a baking sheet and bake for about 15 minutes. Bonus kale chips to enjoy with your breakfast or later as a snack!

Turkey Sausage with Two-Minute Wilted Greens

COMMERCIAL SAUSAGE IS often filled with sugar, the last thing we need first thing in the morning (or ever!). Making your own means you get to be in charge of what goes into it, so you can take charge of your health.

You can make the sausage ahead of time and cook it on the spot. Cook all the patties at once and reheat them throughout the week, or freeze them raw and defrost in the refrigerator the night before you plan to cook them. You could even eat these for dinner in place of your favorite burger recipe! The recipe can be doubled or even tripled.

SERVES 2

12 ounces ground turkey
1 teaspoon dulse granules
1 garlic clove, pressed through a garlic press
¾ teaspoon dried sage
¼ teaspoon dried thyme
¼ teaspoon dried oregano
½ teaspoon plus a pinch of salt
½ teaspoon freshly ground black pepper
Pinch of cayenne pepper (optional)
1 tablespoon coconut oil, extra-virgin olive oil, or ghee
4 kale, collard, or Swiss chard leaves, stemmed, torn into pieces or chopped
2 teaspoons cider vinegar

In a large bowl, combine the turkey, dulse, garlic, sage, thyme, oregano, ¼ teaspoon of the salt, and the black pepper and cayenne, if using. Gently mix with your hands until well combined. Form the mixture into 2½-inch-diameter patties that are about ½ inch thick, to make eight patties.

Melt the oil in a large, nonstick skillet that has a lid over medium heat. Add the patties and cook until well browned, about 5 minutes. Flip and cook until browned on the second side and cooked through. Transfer to plates.

Immediately add the kale to the pan, cover, and cook for 2 minutes, or until wilted. Add the vinegar and pinch of salt and toss with tongs to combine.

Each serving: 44 g protein, 10 g fat, 5 g carbs, 266 calories

(Continues)

**(Turkey Sausage with Two-Minute Wilted
Greens Continued)**

- *Swaps Outs*
  Use beef, pork, or lamb instead of turkey. Omit the oil; you won't need
  it, as the patties will cook in their own fat.

- *Supercharge It!*
  Add a side of sauerkraut (page 174) or kimchi to the plate.

Dilly Smoked Salmon Scramble

SMOKED OR CURED salmon is a treat that adds heart-healthy omega-3
goodness to your morning meal—and it instantly upgrades an everyday
breakfast into something special. You could even serve it for Sunday brunch—
share the Plan Your Plate concept with your guests! If you'd like to add a
starchy carb, a side of a small baked sweet potato (page 180) would be
perfect.

SERVES 2

4 large eggs
1 tablespoon canned unsweetened full-fat coconut milk
¼ teaspoon sea salt
⅛ teaspoon freshly ground black pepper
1 tablespoon extra-virgin olive oil, coconut oil, or ghee
¼ teaspoon ground turmeric
1½ ounces smoked or cured salmon, chopped
1 teaspoon capers
1 tablespoon chopped fresh dill
1 cup mixed salad greens

In a large bowl, beat the eggs with the coconut milk, then beat in the salt
and pepper.

Heat the oil in a large, nonstick skillet over medium heat. Add the turmeric and let it sizzle for about 20 seconds. Add the eggs and fold with a heatproof spatula until set, about 5 minutes. Turn off the heat and fold in the salmon, capers, and dill. Divide between two plates and serve with salad greens alongside.

Each serving: 18 g protein, 20 g fat, 2 g carbs, 260 calories

● *Supercharge It!*
Add a side of Sauerkraut (page 174) to your scramble after it's done (don't heat it, or it will lose its live and active cultures).

TIP: To avoid rubbery eggs, leave the eggs in the pan for a minute before stirring so they begin to set. Then, use a rubber spatula to gently fold the eggs to form curds and continue to fold until there is no more liquidy egg in the pan but the eggs still look fairly wet, about a minute more.

Sesame Asparagus with Fried Eggs

THIS ONE-PAN DISH with a double dose of sesame elevates a simple breakfast to something special. When asparagus isn't in season, try swapping in broccoli or zucchini.

SERVES 2

1 bunch asparagus, woody ends broken off
2 teaspoons toasted sesame oil
½ teaspoon sea salt
¼ teaspoon freshly ground black pepper
1 teaspoon freshly squeezed lemon juice
2 teaspoons coconut oil or ghee
4 large eggs
2 teaspoons toasted sesame seeds

(Continues)

(Sesame Asparagus with Fried Eggs Continued)

In a large skillet with a lid, combine the asparagus, sesame oil, and 1 tablespoon of water. Add ¼ teaspoon of the salt and ⅛ teaspoon of the pepper. Place over medium-high heat and cook, tossing often with tongs, for about 2 minutes, until most of the water is absorbed. Cover and cook for about 5 minutes more, lifting the lid and tossing a couple of times, until the asparagus is crisp-tender and nicely browned in spots. Add the lemon juice, toss, and divide between two plates.

Melt the coconut oil in the same pan and crack the eggs into the pan. Sprinkle with the remaining ¼ teaspoon of salt and the remaining ⅛ teaspoon of pepper, cover, and cook for 3 to 5 minutes, until the eggs are as set or runny as you like. Top the asparagus with the fried eggs, sprinkle with the sesame seeds, and serve.

Each serving: 16 g protein, 20 g fat, 6 g carbs, 263 calories

- **Neglected Veggie Alert!**
  Don't toss out those asparagus ends—toss them into your pot of Bone Broth (page 163) instead. You wouldn't want to miss out on their added flavor and nutrition. Asparagus contains high levels of folate and vitamins A, C, E, and K. It is a natural diuretic that can help fight bloat, and its antioxidant content rivals that of green leafy vegetables. If you're not making bone broth, simply chop the ends, throw them into a small pot, add a couple of cups of water, and simmer for about 20 minutes. Season with salt and enjoy it as a light asparagus sipping broth.

Herb, Shiitake, and Spinach Omelet

IF YOU CAN make scrambled eggs, you can make an omelet (and if it doesn't come out perfect, call it a scramble and no one will be the wiser!). Use this method to make omelets with whatever veggies you have on hand—it's a great way to repurpose leftovers from dinner.

SERVES 2

4 large eggs
2 tablespoons finely chopped fresh parsley or cilantro
¼ teaspoon sea salt
1 tablespoon extra-virgin olive oil or ghee
1 garlic clove, minced
4 shiitake mushrooms, stemmed and finely chopped
⅛ teaspoon ground turmeric
¼ teaspoon freshly ground black pepper
1 cup baby spinach
3 tablespoons Creamy Cashew Cheese (page 170)
1 cup arugula

In a large bowl, beat the eggs, then beat in the parsley and salt.

Heat the oil in a large, nonstick skillet over medium heat. Add the garlic and cook for 30 seconds. Add the mushrooms and cook for about 2 minutes, until softened. Add the turmeric and pepper and cook for 30 seconds, or until aromatic.

Add the eggs to the pan and cook, stirring with a heatproof spatula, for about 30 seconds, until the eggs begin to thicken. Pull the edges of the omelet in toward the center, tilting the pan so the uncooked egg flows to the sides of the pan and underneath the omelet. Cook until just set but still a little wet. Add the spinach to one side of the omelet, cover the pan, and steam until wilted, about 20 seconds. Smear the cheese on the other side of

(Continues)

(Herb, Shitake, and Spinach Omelet Continued)

the omelet and flip one side over the other to close it. Cut in half and serve, with the arugula alongside.

Each serving: 16 g protein, 21 g fat, 8 g carbs, 282 calories

- **Swap Out**
Swap ½ mashed avocado for the Creamy Cashew Cheese.

Very Berry Smoothie Bowl

BLEND FRUIT WITH just a touch of liquid and you get to eat your smoothie with a spoon! Think of it as a dairy- and grain-free version of a yogurt and granola parfait. The bowl is your base, and a sprinkle of crunchy bits—coconut and cacao nibs—is your "cereal" topping. Take charge of your cereal bowl and start the day with multiple superfoods!

SERVES 1

¼ cup almond milk, homemade (page 167) or store-
    bought, plus more if needed
1¼ cups raspberries, blueberries, or strawberries, or a
    combination
½ cup frozen peach or pineapple chunks
1½ tablespoons almond butter, homemade (page 169)
    or store-bought
1 tablespoon canned unsweetened coconut cream or
    coconut milk
1 scoop protein powder
1 teaspoon unsweetened shredded coconut
1 teaspoon raw cacao nibs

Pour the almond milk into a food processor or high-speed blender. Add 1 cup of the raspberries and the peach, almond butter, coconut cream, and protein powder and process until smooth, scraping down the sides if needed. If the consistency is too thin, blend in a couple of ice cubes or more almond milk. Transfer to a bowl, top with the remaining ¼ cup of berries, the coconut, and the cacao nibs, and serve.

Each serving: 21 g protein, 21 g fat, 32 g carbs, 369 calories

● *Swap Out*
Omit the protein powder and include two eggs or 4 ounces of another protein, such as chicken, with your breakfast.

● *Supercharge It!*
Blend a scoop of greens powder into your smoothie bowl.

How to Pick a Protein Powder

Adding protein powder is a quick and easy way of getting a balance of protein into your smoothies and giving yourself an added boost when you're working out. There are many options, but one of my newer favorites is bone broth protein powder, which concentrates the benefits of this liquid superfood (read more about bone broth on page 115) without the dairy, soy, or other legumes found in many protein powders. It also contains collagen and other nutrients to support healthy bones, joints, and cartilage. Choose a bone broth powder that is all natural, from grass-fed animals, with minimal added ingredients, no artificial sweeteners, and at least 20 grams of protein and under 6 grams of carbs per serving. Other dairy- and legume-free protein powder options include collagen, hemp, or egg protein powder. If you're used to using whey protein powder, you'll be avoiding it for just for the ten days. After the ten days, you may try reintroducing it (see page 136).

Carrot Cake Colada Smoothie

TROPICAL COCONUT AND pineapple meet warming carrot cake spices! You'll need to grate the carrot before blending it, to break it down to smoothie consistency. Anti-inflammatory turmeric adds to the golden color of this smoothie and black pepper works to enhance turmeric's health-giving effects. Choose a protein powder that is free of dairy, soy, or other legumes, such as bone broth, collagen, hemp, or egg protein powder (see sidebar, page 191).

SERVES 1

1 cup unsweetened almond milk, homemade (page 167) or
   store-bought
1 scoop protein powder
Pinch of ground nutmeg
1 large carrot, grated
1 teaspoon finely chopped fresh ginger
2 pinches of ground cinnamon
⅛ teaspoon ground turmeric
Pinch of freshly ground black pepper
1 tablespoon no-sugar-added almond butter, homemade (page
   169) or store-bought
2 tablespoons unsweetened coconut cream
½ cup frozen pineapple chunks
4 ice cubes
1 teaspoon unsweetened shredded coconut

In a blender, combine the almond milk, protein powder, nutmeg, carrot, ginger, one pinch of the cinnamon, the turmeric, black pepper, almond butter, coconut cream, pineapple, and ice cubes and blend until smooth. Add a little water if the smoothie is too thick. Pour into a glass, top with the remaining pinch of cinnamon and the shredded coconut, and serve.

Each serving: 19 g protein, 19 g fat, 25 g carbs, 332 calories

- *Swap Out*

Omit the protein powder and instead have two eggs or 4 ounces of another protein such as chicken with your breakfast.

Super Green Smoothie

REMEMBER V3, my challenge of getting more veggies into your day? What better way than first thing in the morning! Lemon juice offsets the bitterness of the greens, and mixed fruit adds sweetness to make it really easy going green. A little avocado goes a long way to thickening your smoothie, and its healthy fats will keep you full through to lunch. Chop and freeze the remaining avocado for future smoothies. Choose a protein powder that is free of dairy, soy, or other legumes, such as bone broth, collagen, hemp, or egg protein powder (see sidebar, page 191).

SERVES 1

2 cups unsweetened almond milk, homemade (page 167) or
  store-bought
1½ tablespoons canned full-fat unsweetened coconut milk
2 teaspoons freshly squeezed lemon juice
1 scoop protein powder
¼ avocado
½ cup frozen raspberries or mixed berries
¼ cup frozen pineapple chunks
2 cups packed spinach or Swiss chard leaves (about 3 ounces)

In a blender, combine all the ingredients and blend until smooth. Pour into a glass and serve.

Each serving: 22 g protein, 19 g fat, 31 g carbs, 359 calories

(Continues)

(Super Green Smoothie Continued)

TIP: *For ease in blending your smoothies, always add liquids to the blender first.*

- **Neglected Veggie Alert!**
Gather cilantro and parsley stems in the freezer and add a handful to your green smoothies.

- **Swap Out**
Omit the protein powder and include two eggs or 4 ounces of another protein such as chicken with your breakfast.

- **Supercharge It!**
Blend in 1 scoop of greens powder.

Coconut Water and Maple Water

Coconut water is the clear liquid you get from cracking open a young coconut. It's an excellent form of hydration, thanks to its high electrolyte, antioxidant, and mineral content (in particular, potassium and magnesium). It's no contest when you compare it to sugar-filled, artificially colored sports drinks. The best coconut water is unpasteurized and unprocessed kind found in the cold case.

Maple water is the sap of the maple tree before it's boiled down to syrup. Packaged maple water is a newcomer to the market, but it's actually been around since the first maple tree was tapped. Like coconut water, it is also rich in electrolytes, antioxidants, and minerals, and it contains about half as much sugar as coconut water and a third of the calories. To give you a picture of how light it is, it takes 10 gallons of maple sap to produce 1 quart of maple syrup!

Both coconut water and maple water are excellent hydration choices for smoothies, straight up as a postworkout thirst quencher, or frozen into ice cubes to add a splash of sweetness to summer coolers.

Cinnamon Chocolate Smoothie

IT TASTES LIKE a milk shake, but you get to drink it for breakfast! A small amount of frozen banana adds body without a ton of sugar, and cinnamon adds blood sugar–regulating effects. Anthocyanins, which give blueberries their brilliant color, add free radical–neutralizing powers. What a great way to start the day! Choose a protein powder that is free of dairy, soy, or legumes, such as bone broth, collagen, hemp, or egg protein powder (see sidebar, page 191).

SERVES 1

- ½ cup unsweetened almond milk, homemade (page 167) or store-bought
- ½ cup coconut water or maple water
- 1½ tablespoons no-sugar-added almond or cashew butter, homemade (page 169) or store-bought
- 2 tablespoons raw cacao powder
- 1 scoop protein powder
- ¼ teaspoon plus a pinch of ground cinnamon
- ⅛ teaspoon almond extract
- Pinch of sea salt
- ¼ cup frozen blueberries
- ½ frozen banana
- 1 teaspoon cacao nibs or chia seeds

In a blender, combine the almond milk, coconut water, almond butter, cacao powder, protein powder, ¼ teaspoon of the cinnamon, the almond extract, salt, blueberries, and banana and blend until smooth. Pour into a glass, sprinkle with the cacao nibs and remaining pinch of cinnamon, and serve.

Each serving: 21 g protein, 18 g fat, 38 g carbs, 377 calories

(Continues)

(Cinnamon Chocolate Smoothie Continued)

- **Swap Out**
  Omit the protein powder and include two eggs or 4 ounces of another protein such as chicken with your breakfast.

- **Supercharge It!**
  Blend a scoop of greens powder into your smoothie.

  TIP: *Keep bananas chunks in the freezer for on-the-spot smoothie making. Half a banana serves as your starchy (fruit) carb for the meal. It's all you need to thicken and sweeten your smoothies without a sugar overload. Feel free to combine banana with berries, as berries are unlimited!*

Lunch

Lemony Kale and Chicken Salad

THE SECRET TO a great kale salad is massaging the leaves before assembling your salad so they're as tender as lettuce. Add chicken and a lot of lemon and you've updated your chicken salad for your unprocessed lifestyle!

SERVES 2

3 tablespoons extra-virgin olive oil
Juice of 1 lemon
1 small garlic clove, pressed through a garlic press
¼ teaspoon sea salt
¼ teaspoon freshly ground black pepper
1 bunch kale, stemmed and finely chopped
10 ounces shredded Poached Chicken (page 178)

In a large bowl, whisk together the oil, lemon juice, garlic, salt, and pepper. Add the kale and massage it into the dressing for about 1 minute. Let stand for 5 minutes. Add the chicken and toss to coat. Divide between two bowls (or containers for lunch boxes) and serve.

Each serving: 45 g protein, 27 g fat, 17 g carbs, 466 calories

- *Supercharge It!*
  - Add 2 teaspoons dulse granules or top with Crunchy Dulse Chips (page 231).
  - Add ½ cup Sauerkraut (page 174) or kimchi.
- *Add V3*
  Try shredded beets, carrots, thinly sliced celery or radishes, or shaved fennel.

Scallion Chicken Salad with No-Peanut Peanut Sauce

DID YOU KNOW that peanuts aren't a nut but a legume? Since we're avoiding legumes, this chicken salad, like a deconstructed spring roll, is slathered with an almond butter sauce that's every bit as tasty as the original. The recipe makes extra sauce for dipping carrot sticks or nori grabbers (page 243) into.

SERVES 2

Chicken Salad
½ cup thinly sliced or shredded cabbage
¼ teaspoon sea salt
½ cup cooked corn kernels
½ cup shredded carrot
½ cup chopped scallions, white and green parts
12 ounces shredded Poached Chicken (page 178)
¼ cup chopped fresh cilantro
6 tablespoons Spicy No-Peanut Peanut Sauce (recipe follows)

(Continues)

(Scallion Chicken Salad Continued)

In a large bowl, toss the cabbage with the salt and massage the cabbage lightly to start to soften it. Add the corn, carrot, and scallions and toss to combine. Add the chicken and cilantro and toss again. Divide between two bowls (or containers for lunch boxes) and top with the sauce.

No-Peanut Peanut Sauce

MAKES ABOUT ¾ CUP

½ cup smooth no-sugar-added almond butter,
　　homemade (page 169) or store-bought
6 tablespoons hot water, or as needed
2 tablespoons coconut aminos
1½ tablespoons freshly squeezed lime juice, or to taste
½ teaspoon red pepper flakes
1 garlic clove, pressed through a garlic press

In a medium-size bowl, whisk together all the ingredients until smooth. Add more water if it's too thick and more lime juice if needed. Store in a covered container in the refrigerator for up to 1 week.

Each serving (chicken salad):
47 g protein, 22 g fat, 22 g carbs, 456 calories
. . .
Each serving (3 tablespoons dressing only):
7 g protein, 18 g fat, 8 g carbs, 201 calories

Thai-Style Shrimp, Cucumber, and Pineapple Salad

WAKE UP YOUR taste buds with clean, bright, fresh flavors! Shrimp adds a subtle sweetness to this salad, so you won't miss the sugar that's sneakily added to many Thai dishes. If you don't have time to poach shrimp, buy precooked shrimp. The salad will keep for up to three days, making it easy to get your lunch ready in advance. Add the herbs just before serving.

SERVES 2

½ English cucumber, peeled and diced
1 cup fresh pineapple chunks
½ red bell pepper, seeded and diced
1 jalapeño chile, thinly sliced (seeded, if you like)
2 tablespoons freshly squeezed lime juice
1 tablespoon Asian fish sauce
¼ cup chopped fresh cilantro
¼ cup chopped fresh mint
1 tablespoon plus ½ teaspoon extra-virgin olive oil
1½ tablespoons raw cashews
Pinch of sea salt

(Continues)

(*Thai-Style Shrimp Salad Continued*)

> 12 ounces Poached Shrimp (page 179)
> 2 lime quarters

In a medium-size bowl, combine the cucumber, pineapple, bell pepper, and jalapeño. Add the lime juice and fish sauce and toss again. Add the cilantro and mint and toss once more. Leave on the counter for 30 minutes to marinate.

Heat ½ teaspoon of the oil in a small skillet over medium heat. Add the cashews and pinch of salt and toast, stirring constantly, for 3 to 5 minutes, until lightly browned. Transfer to a plate and allow to cool.

Divide the salad between two bowls (or containers for lunch boxes) and top with the shrimp. Drizzle the remaining 1 tablespoon of oil on top, sprinkle with the cashews, and serve.

Each serving: 33 g protein, 13 g fat, 22 g carbs, 332 calories

- *Add V3*
Serve on a bed of Cauliflower Rice (page 176) or Zucchini Noodles (page 217).

Mango, Avocado, and Arugula Shrimp Salad

THE SALAD IS tangy, creamy, and a little sweet. Mango adds its perfumy flavor and more vitamin C than an orange! Look for fish sauce with Thai ingredients; choose one that is sugar-free, such as Red Boat brand.

SERVES 2

> ½ ripe mango, cut into ½-inch cubes
> ½ avocado, cut into ¼-inch cubes
> ½ small red bell pepper, seeded and cut into ¼-inch cubes
> ½ jalapeño chile, sliced (seeded, if you like)

¼ cup chopped fresh scallions, white and green parts
¼ cup chopped fresh basil
1½ tablespoons freshly squeezed lime juice
1 tablespoon Asian fish sauce
12 ounces Poached Shrimp (page 179)
4 cups arugula

In a medium-size bowl, combine the mango, avocado, bell pepper, jalapeño, scallions, and basil and toss to combine. Add the lime juice and fish sauce and toss again. Add the shrimp and toss once more. Divide the arugula between two bowls (or containers for lunch boxes) and top with the shrimp salad.

Each serving: 34 g protein, 10 g fat, 25 g carbs, 316 calories

• *Swap Outs*
  • Shredded chicken for the shrimp
  • Pineapple for the mango
  • Cilantro for the basil
  • Red onion for the scallions

TIP: *Mango works well in both sweet and savory dishes. Try it Mexican style, sprinkled with salt, chili powder, and lime juice!*

Tahini Tuna Salad

TAHINI (SESAME PASTE) is what gives body to hummus, and it provides creaminess to this classic tuna salad. And it joins forces with the tuna for a double hit of omega-3 fatty acids to feed your brain and heart. The minerals magnesium and phosphorus contained in the sesame seeds help improve bone density.

SERVES 2

(Continues)

(Tahini Tuna Salad Continued)

3 tablespoons tahini
    1 tablespoon freshly squeezed lemon juice, or to taste
    ¼ teaspoon garlic powder
    ⅛ teaspoon celery seeds
    ½ teaspoon sea salt
    ¼ teaspoon freshly ground black pepper
    2 (5-ounce) cans water-packed tuna
    2 tablespoons minced celery
    2 tablespoons minced carrot
    2 tablespoons minced red onion
    1 tablespoon capers
    1 tablespoon chopped fresh flat-leaf parsley
    2 cups mixed lettuce leaves
    ½ cucumber, thinly sliced

In a small bowl, whisk together the tahini, 3 tablespoons of water, and the lemon juice. Add a little more water if the dressing is too thick. Whisk in the garlic powder, celery seeds, salt, and pepper.

Drain the tuna, put it in a large bowl, and break it up with a fork. Add the celery, carrot, red onion, capers, and parsley. Add the dressing and stir to combine. Taste and add more lemon juice if needed. Arrange the lettuce and cucumber on two plates (or containers for lunch boxes), top with the tuna mixture, and serve.

Each serving: 39 g protein, 15 g fat, 13 g carbs, 337 calories

• Supercharge It!

Serve with a side of Sauerkraut (page 174) or a naturally fermented dill pickle. Or tear a sheet of nori and add it to the bowl for a naturally salty, crisp finish.

TIP: To add a carb element, serve with a small sweet potato or white potato on the side or chopped and added as the base of the salad.

Sea Vegetable Shrimp Lettuce Wraps

ARAME, A STRANDLIKE sea vegetable with a mild, sweet flavor, is a great choice for seaweed newbies looking to reap the incredible detoxifying benefits of this chlorophyll-rich food. Read more about this superfood on page 108. If you're packing your wraps to go, put the lettuce leaves in a separate container so they stay crisp until you're ready to eat.

SERVES 2

¼ cup arame
1½ tablespoons toasted sesame oil
1 large yellow onion, sliced into half moons
1 garlic clove, minced
1 teaspoon minced fresh ginger
1 large carrot, cut into thin matchsticks
1 tablespoon coconut aminos
2 teaspoons freshly squeezed lemon juice
6 romaine lettuce leaves
12 ounces Poached Shrimp (page 179)
1 tablespoon toasted sesame seeds
Large pinch of sea salt

Put the arame in a large bowl and add warm water to cover by a couple of inches. Let sit for 10 minutes, then drain.

Heat 1 tablespoon of the oil in a large skillet over medium heat. Add the onion and cook until softened and starting to brown, about 10 minutes. Add the garlic and ginger and cook for 1 minute, or until aromatic. Add the carrot and cook until it is softened but still holds its shape, about 3 minutes. If the mixture looks a little dry or sticks to the pan, add a splash of water. Add the drained arame and cook for about 2 minutes to soften it. Add the coconut aminos and cook for 20 seconds. Turn off the heat and stir in the lemon juice.

(Continues)

(Sea Vegetable Shrimp Lettuce Wraps)

Divide the lettuce leaves between two plates. Spoon the arame mixture on top and add the shrimp. Drizzle with the remaining ½ tablespoon of the oil, top with the sesame seeds and salt, and serve.

Each serving: 33 g protein, 15 g fat, 21 g carbs, 345 calories

TIP: Use the mineral-rich water from soaking the arame to water your plants.

Citrus Tuna Poke Bowl

POKE (PRONOUNCED POH-KAY) is a raw fish salad from Hawaii that's typically marinated in soy sauce. Here we swap in coconut aminos to avoid the added estrogen associated with soy and add lime juice for extra zing. Poke is supersimple to put together and is especially refreshing when it's hot out. Since you'll be eating the fish raw, make sure to purchase sushi-grade tuna (ask at the fish counter to be sure).

SERVES 2

2½ tablespoons coconut aminos, or to taste
1 tablespoon freshly squeezed lime juice, or to taste
1 tablespoon toasted sesame oil
1 large orange
12 ounces best-quality tuna, cut into ½-inch cubes
3 scallions, thinly sliced
1 serrano or other chile, thinly sliced
3 cups raw Cauliflower Rice (page 176; optional), for serving
½ seedless cucumber, thinly sliced
½ small avocado, cut into small cubes
1 teaspoon toasted sesame seeds

In a large bowl, whisk together the coconut aminos, lime juice, and sesame oil. Zest the orange directly over the bowl and whisk in the zest. Cut the orange into segments (see sidebar), then chop the segments. Add the segments and any orange juice you squeezed from the fruit along the way. Add the tuna, scallions, and chile and toss to mix well. Let sit on the counter for up to 30 minutes or in the refrigerator for up to 2 hours, tossing to distribute the seasonings every so often. Just before serving, toss, then taste and add more coconut aminos or lime juice, if needed.

If you're including the cauliflower rice, divide it between two bowls (or containers for lunch boxes). Top with the cucumber, followed by the tuna mixture, avocado, and sesame seeds.

Each serving (without optional cauliflower):
49 g protein, 17 g fat, 34 g carbs, 470 calories

- *Swap Outs*
  - Salmon for the tuna
  - Mayonnaise (make sure it's made with extra-virgin olive oil or avocado oil, not soybean oil) for the avocado as your fat (top each bowl with 1 tablespoon)

- *Supercharge It!*
  Garnish your bowls with toasted nori slices for a deconstructed sushi effect. The nori will add crunch and metabolism-stimulating iodine.

How to Segment Citrus

Cut a slice from the top and bottom of the orange, grapefruit, or other citrus fruit to reveal the flesh. Stand the fruit upright and slice off the peel from the sides in wide strips, cutting downward, following the shape of the fruit to remove all of the white pith. Hold the fruit over a bowl and use a sharp paring knife to cut along both sides of each segment, releasing the segments and allowing them and the juice to drop into the bowl beneath. The fancy term for this technique is to *supreme*. Remove the seeds as you go and squeeze any remaining juice from the pith into the bowl.

Spicy Sausage, Pepper, and Onion Bowl

THE INGREDIENTS READ a little like a sub sandwich . . . but the recipe subs out the bread for lots of veggies, including free radical–fighting and fiber-filled fennel. Look for no-sugar-added turkey sausage, such as a brand that's labeled "paleo style."

SERVES 2

2 tablespoons extra-virgin olive oil or coconut oil
10 ounces turkey sausage links, sliced ½ inch thick
1 medium-size yellow onion, thinly sliced
1 medium-size red bell pepper, seeded and thinly sliced
1 small fennel bulb, cored, fronds chopped and reserved,
    thinly sliced
2 garlic cloves, minced
1 teaspoon dried oregano
½ teaspoon red pepper flakes
1 cup prepared no-sugar-added tomato sauce
¼ teaspoon sea salt, or to taste

In a large skillet, heat 1 tablespoon of the oil over medium heat. Add the sausage and cook until browned on the bottom, 3 to 5 minutes, then flip and cook until browned on the second side, another 3 to 5 minutes. Transfer from the pan to a plate.

Add the remaining 1 tablespoon of the oil to the pan. Add the onion, bell pepper, and fennel and cook until softened and starting to brown, about 10 minutes. Add the garlic and cook for about 1 minute, until aromatic. Add the oregano and red pepper flakes and cook for 1 minute. Add the tomato sauce, bring to a simmer, and cook for 10 minutes. Add the sausage and cook to heat through. Stir in the reserved fennel fronds and serve.

Each serving: 29 g protein, 30 g fat, 25 g carbs, 467 calories

- *Add V3*
Serve with a side of Cauliflower Rice (page 176).

Simplest Taco Salad Bowl

WITH CHICKEN AND salsa on hand, this recipe involves little more than tossing and serving. To make it even easier, use a store-bought salsa, but check the label closely to make sure it contains no sugar or artificial ingredients.

SERVES 2

12 ounces shredded Poached Chicken (page 178)
1 cup Green Salsa (page 173) or store-bought green or red salsa
3 cups chopped romaine lettuce or shredded cabbage
½ avocado, finely chopped
¼ cup chopped fresh cilantro
1 lime, cut in half

In a large bowl, combine the chicken and salsa and toss to coat the chicken in the salsa. Divide the lettuce between two bowls (or containers for lunch boxes) and top with the avocado and cilantro. Serve with a lime half for squeezing.

Each serving: 41 g protein, 13 g fat, 19 g carbs, 347 calories

Pesto Turkey Burgers

BURGERS—MINUS THE BUNS—are a great friend to fat loss and a busy lifestyle, as it's easy to make them in advance and simply reheat when you're ready to eat. And a little pesto is all it takes to upgrade an ordinary burger to out-of-this-world delicious! Choose the crispiest lettuce you can find—one that will hold the shape of a burger, such as Bibb or butter lettuce. To add a starchy carb, serve with a small sweet potato or white potato alongside each burger.

(Continues)

(Pesto Turkey Burgers Continued)

Cook only as many burgers as you're going to serve; if you're not cooking all the patties at once, refrigerate or freeze the raw patties until you're ready to cook them. These don't freeze well after they are cooked.

SERVES 6

2 pounds ground turkey, preferably dark meat
1 cup chopped fresh cilantro or basil, or a combination
4 garlic cloves, pressed through a garlic press
2 teaspoons coconut aminos
1 teaspoon sea salt
1 tablespoon extra-virgin olive oil or coconut oil
6 very crisp lettuce leaves
6 thick tomato slices
½ cup Loaded Greens Pesto (page 172)

In a large bowl, gently mix the turkey, cilantro, garlic, coconut aminos, and salt until just combined. Do not overwork the meat, or it will become tough. Form into six loosely packed patties.

Heat the oil in a large skillet over medium heat. Add three of the patties and cook until browned and cooked through, 5 to 6 minutes per side. Transfer the burgers to a plate and cook the remaining patties in the same way.

Assemble your burgers by slipping each into a lettuce leaf, topping with a tomato slice, and finishing with a heaping tablespoon of pesto.

Each serving: 33 g protein, 20 g fat, 4 g carbs, 318 calories

- Swaps Outs
  - Trade the turkey for ground beef, pork, or lamb. Cut the oil for cooking in half.
  - Go traditional by swapping the pesto for no-sugar-added ketchup. For your fat, enjoy ¼ avocado for each serving.

Dinner

Chicken and Spinach Loaded Sweet Potatoes

YOU DON'T NEED sour cream and cheese to load your potatoes! Swap in protein-rich chicken and spinach and this bar food becomes a balanced meal that's every bit as comforting as the original.

SERVES 2

2 large Baked Sweet Potatoes (page 180)
1 tablespoon extra-virgin olive oil, coconut oil, or ghee
1 garlic clove, minced
2 cups baby spinach
8 ounces Poached Chicken (page 178), shredded
¼ teaspoon ground cinnamon
¼ teaspoon sea salt
¼ teaspoon freshly ground black pepper
1 tablespoon toasted slivered almonds
1 tablespoon pomegranate seeds (optional)

Cut the sweet potatoes in half and remove most of their flesh, leaving a little at the bottom of the jacket. Reserve half of the flesh for another use. Coarsely mash the remaining sweet potato flesh.

In a medium-size skillet, heat the oil. Add the garlic and cook for about 1 minute, until aromatic. Add the spinach and stir until wilted, about 1 minute. Add the chicken, cinnamon, salt, and pepper and stir until heated through. Scoop the mixture into the four sweet potato shells, top with the slivered almonds and pomegranate seeds, if using, and serve.

Each serving:
29 g protein, 11 g fat, 22 g carbs, 306 calories

Oven-Baked Hot Wings and Sweet Potatoes

LOW AND SLOW, followed by some time at high heat is the secret to super-crispy wings straight from the oven. The starting low temperature begins to dry the wings out and melt away their fat, which then crisps up when you raise the heat. With all that time you'll save on prep, go ahead and take some time for yourself while you're waiting for them to be done: do a workout, kick back with a book, or take a nice long bath.

SERVES 2

Coconut oil cooking spray
1 pound chicken wings
½ teaspoon sea salt
2 tablespoons hot sauce, plus more to taste
2 small (2-ounce) Baked Sweet Potatoes (page 180)

Preheat the oven to 250°F. Line a baking sheet with parchment paper and coat the sheet with cooking spray.

Pat dry the wings of excess moisture with paper towels. Place in a bowl and toss with the salt. Arrange the wings in a single layer on the prepared pan. Bake for 45 minutes. Increase the heat to 425°F and bake for another 45 minutes, or until the wings are browned and crispy. Place in a bowl along with their juices and toss with the hot sauce to coat. Serve with the baked sweet potatoes.

Each serving: 27 g protein, 18 g fat, 13 g carbs, 325 calories

- *Add V3*
Serve with lots of salad greens.

One-Pan Chicken Fajitas

NOT JUST FOR eating out! While it might not have the dramatic flair of the sizzling hot pan, this version of fajitas tastes every bit as amazing. Ten minutes prep followed by twenty minutes in the oven, all in one pan, and they're done. You can't beat that!

SERVES 2

1 teaspoon chili powder

1 teaspoon paprika

1 teaspoon sea salt

1 teaspoon freshly ground black pepper

1 small red bell pepper, seeded and cut into ½-inch-thick strips

1 small green bell pepper, seeded and cut into ½-inch-thick strips

1 small yellow bell pepper, seeded and cut into ½-inch-thick strips

1 medium-size yellow onion, cut in half and sliced

10 ounces boneless, skinless chicken breast, sliced into ½-inch-thick strips

1 garlic clove, minced

1½ tablespoons extra-virgin olive oil

1½ tablespoons freshly squeezed lime juice

¼ cup chopped fresh cilantro

¼ small avocado, diced

Preheat the oven to 400°F. Line a baking sheet with parchment paper.
In a small bowl, mix together the chili powder, paprika, salt, and pepper. Spread the bell peppers and onion over the prepared baking sheet. Top with the chicken, then sprinkle the garlic and seasoning mixture evenly over the chicken strips. Drizzle the oil on top and toss to coat the ingredients in the oil and spices. Spread out the ingredients in an even layer and bake, tossing once halfway through, until the vegetables are softened and the chicken is cooked through, about 20 minutes. Drizzle the lime juice over the top, sprinkle with the cilantro, and serve garnished with the avocado.

Each serving: 31 g protein, 18 g fat, 17 g carbs, 347 calories

Turkey Tacos

A THANKSGIVING BINGE on turkey can make us overly sleepy, but in everyday meal servings, the tryptophan contained in the bird helps improve overall sleep quality. And as turkey contains metabolism-supporting selenium and is high in protein and low in calories, it can play an important part in unprocessing your diet. So, bring on turkey taco night, and lighten it up with lettuce leaf taco shells!

SERVES 2

- 2 teaspoons extra-virgin olive oil, coconut oil, or ghee
- 2 garlic cloves, finely chopped
- 12 ounces ground turkey
- 2 teaspoons chili powder
- 1 teaspoon dulse granules
- ½ teaspoon paprika
- ¼ teaspoon ground turmeric
- ¼ teaspoon freshly ground black pepper
- ½ teaspoon plus a pinch of sea salt
- 4 shiitake mushrooms, stemmed and finely chopped
- 1 teaspoon cider vinegar
- 6 romaine lettuce leaves
- ½ avocado, diced

Heat the oil in a large skillet over medium heat. Add the garlic and cook for 1 minute, or until aromatic. Add the turkey, chili powder, dulse, paprika, turmeric, pepper, and ½ teaspoon of the salt. Cook, breaking up the meat with a wooden spoon, until it is cooked through and no longer pink, about 15 minutes. Add the mushrooms and cook for about 5 minutes, until cooked through. Turn off the heat and add the vinegar. Allow to cool slightly, then divide the turkey among the lettuce leaves, top with the avocado and a pinch of salt, and serve.

Each serving: 45 g protein, 15 g fat, 12 g carbs, 337 calories

- *Add V3*
Double the lettuce leaves to make thicker, more veggie-full tacos.

Smoky Chocolate Turkey Chili

COCOA POWDER ADDS deep flavor to this no-bean chili, and chipotle gives it a blast of smoky heat. That's my kind of comfort food! Although the ingredient list is a little long, the method is simple and it's all done in one pot. Make sure to cook the chili the full hour to allow the flavors to develop. Freeze single-serving portions for multiple lunches or dinners.

SERVES 6

- 2 tablespoons extra-virgin olive oil, coconut oil, or ghee
- 2 medium-size white onions, finely chopped
- 3 garlic cloves, minced
- 2 pounds ground turkey
- 2 tablespoons tomato paste
- 2 tablespoons raw cacao powder
- 2 tablespoons chili powder
- 1 tablespoon chipotle chile powder
- 2 teaspoons dried oregano
- 2 teaspoons ground cumin
- ¼ teaspoon ground allspice
- ½ teaspoon ground turmeric
- ½ teaspoon freshly ground black pepper
- 2 teaspoons dulse granules
- 2 teaspoons sea salt
- 1 (14.5-ounce) can diced tomatoes, with juices
- 1 cup Bone Broth (page 163)
- 1 medium-size sweet potato, cut into 1-inch cubes
- 1 cup fresh or frozen and thawed corn kernels
- 1 tablespoon cider vinegar

TOPPINGS:
Chopped avocado (1 tablespoon per serving)
Finely chopped white onion
Chopped fresh cilantro

(Continues)

(Smoky Chocolate Turkey Chile Continued)

Heat the oil in a large saucepan over medium heat. Add the onions and cook until softened and translucent, about 10 minutes. Add the garlic and cook for about 1 minute, until fragrant. Add the ground turkey, breaking it up with a wooden spoon, and cook until starting to brown, about 10 minutes. Add the tomato paste and cook for 2 minutes. Combine the cacao powder, chili powder, chipotle chile powder, oregano, cumin, allspice, turmeric, black pepper, dulse flakes, and salt in a small bowl. Add the spice mixture to the turkey mixture and stir well to work it into the meat. Add the tomatoes, broth, and sweet potato and bring to a simmer. Lower the heat to maintain a gentle simmer and cook for 1 hour. Add the corn kernels and cook for about 1 minute to heat through. Add the vinegar, taste, and adjust the seasonings if needed. Serve topped with chopped avocado, white onion, and cilantro.

Each serving: 42 g protein, 9 g fat, 23 g carbs, 327 calories

- *Swap Outs*
  - Omit the sweet potato or corn to lower the carb content of your chili.
  - Use beef, pork, or lamb instead of the turkey; reduce the oil to 1 tablespoon.
  - Use smoked paprika instead of chipotle chile powder for a milder chili.

Seared Scallops and Turmeric Cauliflower Rice

SCALLOPS TEND TO intimidate many people, but they are in fact super-easy to make and go from pan to plate in under five minutes. Just follow the instructions carefully, flipping each scallop in the order you added them and avoid overcooking them, and your scallops will come out buttery, not rubbery, every time. It will be like a five-star restaurant meal in the comfort of your home!

SERVES 2

12 ounces scallops
2 tablespoons ghee or coconut oil
1 small onion, finely chopped
1 garlic clove, minced
¼ teaspoon ground turmeric
2 cups raw Cauliflower Rice (page 176)
½ teaspoon sea salt
½ teaspoon freshly ground black pepper
1 tablespoon dried currants
1 tablespoon chopped fresh parsley, dill, or cilantro

Rinse the scallops under cold water and pat dry with paper towels. Place the scallops on a plate and let them come to room temperature while you make the cauliflower rice.

In a large skillet, heat 1 tablespoon of the ghee over medium heat. Add the onion and cook until softened, about 5 minutes. Add the garlic and cook for about 1 minute, until fragrant. Add the turmeric and cook for 30 seconds. Add the cauliflower rice, ¼ teaspoon of the salt, and ¼ teaspoon of the pepper and cook for another 5 minutes, or until the cauliflower rice is crisp-tender. Stir in the currants and parsley and divide the cauliflower rice between two plates.

Wipe out the pan, increase the heat to medium-high, and add the remaining 1 tablespoon of ghee. Sprinkle the scallops with ⅛ teaspoon of the salt and ⅛ teaspoon of the pepper. Add the scallops, working around the pan like the hands of a clock and adding the first scallop at the twelve o'clock spot. Sprinkle with the remaining ⅛ teaspoon of salt and the remaining ⅛ teaspoon of pepper. Cook for about 2 minutes, until lightly browned on the bottom. Flip the scallops, starting at twelve o'clock, and cook until lightly browned on the second side and white and tender inside, another 1 to 2 minutes. Arrange the scallops over the cauliflower rice and serve.

(Continues)

(Seared Scallops and Turmeric Cauliflower Rice Continued)

Each serving: 24 g protein, 16 g fat, 21 g carbs, 322 calories

- **Add V3**
  Add Swiss chard or another tender green to the pan after you remove
  the scallops. Cover and cook until wilted, season with salt and pepper,
  and serve on the side.

Baked Whitefish with Green Salsa and Fresh Corn

TANGY GREEN SALSA stands out against the sweet, mild flavor of whitefish. This recipe is really simple to make; to make it even simpler, use a prepared all-natural, sugar-free salsa.

SERVES 2

1 cup Green Salsa (page 173)
2 (6-ounce) white fish fillets, such as halibut, flounder, bass, or
   cod
1½ tablespoons ghee, melted and cooled
½ teaspoon plus a pinch of sea salt
¼ teaspoon freshly ground black pepper
1½ tablespoons pumpkin seeds
2 small ears of corn, cooked

Preheat the oven to 400°F.

Spread a thin layer of the salsa into a baking pan large enough to hold
both of the fish fillets. Set the fish fillets into the baking pan, brush with
1 tablespoon of the ghee, and sprinkle with ½ teaspoon of the salt and the
pepper. Pour the rest of the salsa over the fish. Place in the oven and bake for
about 10 minutes, until the fish flakes easily with a fork. Remove from the

oven, divide the fish and salsa between two plates, and top with the pumpkin seeds. Spread the remaining ½ tablespoon of ghee over the corn, sprinkle the corn with a pinch of salt, and serve.

Each serving: 37 g protein, 19 g fat, 23 g carbs, 397 calories

● *Add V3*
Serve on a bed of very thinly sliced cabbage.

Zucchini Noodles and Shrimp with Loaded Greens Pesto

YOU WON'T MISS the pasta when you load your plate with 100 percent vegetable noodles. The neutral flavor of zucchini takes well to any pasta sauce you please, from tomato to garlic and olive oil and pesto.

SERVES 2

2 medium-size zucchini
12 ounces large shrimp, peeled and deveined
½ teaspoon sea salt
¼ teaspoon freshly ground black pepper, plus more for sprinkling
1 tablespoon extra-virgin olive oil
1 medium-size tomato, chopped
¼ cup Loaded Greens Pesto (page 172)

To make the zucchini noodles, use a spiral vegetable slicer or vegetable peeler to cut the zucchini into spaghetti-shape noodles. Stop when you reach the seeds in the middle. Wrap the noodles in paper towels to remove some of their moisture while you make the shrimp (you can do this up to 1 hour in advance).

Rinse the shrimp and pat dry with paper towels. Toss with ¼ teaspoon of the salt and the pepper.

(Continues)

(Zuccinni Noodles and Shrimp Loaded with Greens Pesto Continued)

Heat the oil in large skillet over medium-high heat. Treating the skillet as the face of a clock, add the shrimp one by one, starting at twelve o'clock, and cook until the shrimp start to turn pink, about 2 minutes. Using tongs, turn the shrimp in the order you placed them in the pan and cook until the second side starts to turn pink and the shrimp is almost cooked through, about another 2 minutes. Transfer the shrimp to a bowl, leaving their juices in the pan. Add the zucchini noodles and tomatoes to the pan and toss with tongs until the noodles and tomatoes are slightly softened, about 3 minutes. Transfer to the bowl, add the pesto (and a little water to loosen it if necessary) and the remaining ¼ teaspoon of salt, and gently toss to combine. Spoon into bowls and serve with a sprinkle of pepper.

Each serving: 34 g protein, 28 g fat, 13 g carbs, 426 calories

● **Neglected Veggie Alert!**
Add the seedy core of the zucchini to your Bone Broth (page 163) or chop it finely and add it to tomato sauce, chili, or chicken soup.

Garlicky Shrimp, Shiitake, and Broccoli Stir-fry

GINGER, GARLIC, AND scallions—the holy trinity of Chinese food—provide the flavor base for this satisfying stir-fry. And it comes together in just ten minutes! Don't forget to save the broccoli stems—peel and chop this neglected veggie and add it to the pan along with the florets.

SERVES 2

1½ tablespoons coconut aminos
1 tablespoon white wine vinegar

1½ teaspoons toasted sesame oil
    1 teaspoon water
    3 garlic cloves, pressed through a garlic press
    1½ teaspoons minced fresh ginger
    ½ teaspoon red pepper flakes
    12 ounces large shrimp, peeled and deveined
    ¼ teaspoon sea salt
    1 tablespoon extra-virgin olive oil, coconut oil, or ghee
    1 small head broccoli, cut into small florets
    4 shiitake mushrooms, stemmed and chopped
    1 scallion, white and green parts, thinly sliced
    2 cups Cauliflower Rice (page 176; optional)
    1½ tablespoons toasted slivered almonds

In a small bowl, whisk together the coconut aminos, vinegar, toasted sesame oil, water, garlic, ginger, and red pepper flakes.

Rinse the shrimp and pat dry with paper towels. Toss with the salt.

Heat 1½ teaspoons of the olive oil in large skillet over medium-high heat. Treating the skillet as the face of a clock, add the shrimp one by one, starting at twelve o'clock, and cook until the shrimp start to turn pink, about 2 minutes. Using tongs, turn the shrimp in the order you placed them in the pan and cook until the second side starts to turn pink and the shrimp is almost cooked through, about another 2 minutes. Transfer the shrimp to a bowl along with their juices.

Add the remaining 1½ teaspoons of olive oil to the same pan. Add the broccoli and mushrooms and cook, stirring often, until the vegetables are crisp-tender, 3 to 5 minutes. Return the shrimp to the pan along with its juices. Whisk the coconut aminos mixture, add it to the pan, and cook, stirring constantly, until the vegetables and shrimp are cooked through, about 1 minute. Stir in the scallions. Serve, over cauliflower rice, if you like, topped with the almonds.

Each serving: 36 g protein, 16 g fat, 21 g carbs, 362 calories

(Continues)

(*Garlicky Shrimp, Shiitake, and Broccoli Stir-fry* Continued)

- **Add V3**
Top with a generous garnish of broccoli sprouts or other sprouts.

TIP: *Save the peels from unpeeled shrimp. Put them in a pot with a quart of bone broth. Bring to a simmer, cook for 30 minutes, then strain and sip on the shrimp-flavored broth or use it in your recipes.*

Broiled Salmon with Blackened Scallions and Loaded Greens Pesto

WHEN IT COMES to salmon, less is more. Almost no work at all rewards you with a really tasty meal. With Loaded Greens Pesto handy in the freezer, dinner is just a trip to the fish counter away.

SERVES 2

1 bunch scallions, ends trimmed
1 tablespoon extra-virgin olive oil or ghee
½ teaspoon plus a pinch of sea salt
2 (6-ounce) wild salmon fillets, 1 to 1½ inches thick
2 teaspoons freshly squeezed lemon juice
¼ teaspoon freshly ground black pepper
3 tablespoons Loaded Greens Pesto (page 172)

Preheat the broiler. Line a rimmed baking sheet with foil. Place the scallions on the prepared baking sheet, toss with 1 teaspoon of the oil and a pinch of the salt, and broil until lightly charred, about 3 minutes. Transfer the scallions from the pan to two plates.

Place the fish, skin side down, in a single layer on the same pan. Brush with the remaining 2 teaspoons of oil and the lemon juice and sprinkle with the salt and pepper. Broil until the fish is just opaque in the center, about 8 minutes.

Serve the fish with the pesto and scallions.

Each serving: 36 g protein, 27 g fat, 5 g carbs, 402 calories

● *Add V3*

Top with some beautiful microgreens or baby arugula.

TIP: When scallions are roasted, they're way more than a garnish. You'll have no problem finishing off a bunch. What a great way to get in your V3!

Why You Should Go Wild

If you're concerned about the mercury levels in fish, pass on farmed salmon and go wild. Wild salmon has been found to have much lower levels of mercury, safe enough that you can eat it on a regular basis. Wild salmon also has half the fat of farmed salmon. But if we're not fearing fat, why does that matter? Because in the case of salmon, fat-soluble toxins such as PCBs (a banned chemical that's also found in asbestos) can accumulate in that fat. What's more, farmed salmon live in overcrowded nets, where disease can easily spread. While wild salmon swim free and easy, farmed salmon are vaccinated and fed antibiotics to prevent them from getting sick. If farmed salmon looks as good as wild, don't be fooled. Farmed salmon is often fed artificial dyes to give it that vibrant salmon color that wild salmon get from eating their natural seafood diet.

Soups and Salad

Hot and Sour Egg Drop Soup

THIS SPICY, SOUR comfort food soup combines the best of two classics. It is at its height served just after cooking; consider making a half recipe if there are just two of you, or to turn it into a meal for two, serve double portions with a protein, such as shrimp, added at the end, and an avocado garnish.

SERVES 4

4 cups Bone Broth (page 163)
1 celery rib, including leaves, thinly sliced
1 teaspoon red pepper flakes
4 shiitake mushrooms, stemmed and thinly sliced
3 tablespoons coconut aminos
¼ teaspoon sea salt, or to taste
2 large eggs, beaten
¼ cup cider vinegar
1 teaspoon toasted sesame oil
1 scallion, white and green parts, thinly sliced

Bring the broth to a boil in a medium-size saucepan over high heat. Add the celery and red pepper flakes, lower the heat to medium, and cook for 1 minute. Add the mushrooms and cook for another minute, or until the celery is crisp-tender and the mushrooms are softened. Lower the heat to maintain a bare simmer. Add the coconut aminos and salt and cook for 1 minute. Slowly pour the beaten egg into the broth in a thin, steady stream. Let the egg set for 15 seconds, then stir to gently incorporate it. Remove from the heat and stir in the vinegar and oil. Taste and add more salt if needed, then add the scallion. Spoon into cups and serve.

Each serving: 14 g protein, 4 g fat, 7 g carbs, 122 calories

● *Add V3*
Add extra veggies, such as spinach or Swiss chard.

Soothing Butternut Squash Soup

SQUASH BECOMES SUPERCREAMY when blended, so you don't need to add dairy to make a thick, comforting pot of squash soup. Warming ginger helps burn body fat, and cinnamon gives a sweet taste while helping to control blood sugar. This soup freezes well, so you can have a bowl now and save some for later. You may swap in kabocha, Hubbard, or another winter squash depending on availability.

SERVES 6 (MAKES ABOUT 8 CUPS)

1 tablespoon extra-virgin olive oil, coconut oil, or ghee
1 medium-size yellow onion, finely chopped
2 garlic cloves, minced
1 tablespoon minced fresh ginger
½ teaspoon ground cinnamon
½ teaspoon ground turmeric
½ teaspoon freshly ground black pepper
¼ teaspoon ground allspice
¼ teaspoon paprika
Pinch of cayenne pepper
3 cups chopped butternut squash (1½-inch cubes, from about a
    2-pound squash, or a 20-ounce package chopped squash)
1 large carrot, chopped
6 cups Bone Broth (page 163)
1 teaspoon sea salt, or to taste
2 teaspoons freshly squeezed lemon juice, or to taste

Heat the oil in a large saucepan over medium heat. Add the onion and cook until softened, about 5 minutes. Add the garlic and ginger and cook until softened and the onion is starting to brown, another 2 minutes. Add the cinnamon, turmeric, black pepper, allspice, paprika, and cayenne and cook for 1 minute, or until aromatic.

(Continues)

(Soothing Butternut Squash Soup Continued)

Add the squash, carrot, broth, and salt, increase the heat to high, and bring to a simmer. Lower the heat to maintain a simmer and cook for about 30 minutes, until the squash and carrot are softened. Working in two batches, transfer the soup to a blender and blend until smooth. Add the lemon juice, taste, and adjust the seasonings with more salt and/or lemon juice if needed. Spoon into bowls and serve. The soup will keep for up to 5 days in the refrigerator or in the freezer for up to 2 months.

Each serving: 11 g protein, 3 g fat, 13 g carbs, 116 calories

- **Supercharge It!**
Top with Crunchy Dulse Chips (page 231).

TIP: For extra creaminess, stir in a little coconut milk or coconut cream near the end of cooking.

Tomato, Zucchini, and Basil Soup

TOMATO SOUP DOESN'T need dairy to give it a creamy texture. In this soup, zucchini is blended in to create a 100 percent clean vegetable cream base. Serve as a starter or enjoy it in mugs as a between-meal snack.

SERVES 2

1 tablespoon extra-virgin olive oil, ghee, or coconut oil
1 large onion, chopped
2 garlic cloves, chopped
1 teaspoon dried oregano
½ teaspoon freshly ground black pepper
¼ teaspoon ground turmeric
1 (14-ounce) can diced tomatoes
2 cups Bone Broth (page 163)
½ teaspoon sea salt, or to taste

1 medium-size zucchini, chopped
1 tablespoon cider vinegar
¼ cup chopped fresh basil

In a large saucepan, heat the oil over medium heat. Add the onion and cook for about 7 minutes, until softened and starting to brown. Add the garlic and cook for about 1 minute, until aromatic. Add the oregano, pepper, and turmeric and cook for 30 seconds. Add the tomatoes with their juices, the bone broth, and salt and bring to a simmer. Lower the heat to maintain a simmer and cook for 20 minutes to blend the flavors. Add the zucchini and cook for about 10 minutes, until softened. Remove from the heat and add the vinegar. Transfer to a blender and blend until smooth. Add the basil and pulse to combine. If the mixture is too thick, thin it with a little bone broth or water. Pour into bowls or mugs for sipping and serve.

Each serving: 14 g protein, 8 g fat, 23 g carbs, 213 calories

Neglected Veggie Stem Soup

NOTHING GOES TO waste in this soup! Save your stems from herbs, mushrooms, and other veggies to flavor your broth and give it a nutritional boost. Use this recipe as a base, and see my list of Neglected Veggies on pages 111 to 112 for more ideas. This soup is best sipped by the mugful and it doubles or triples easily based on what you have on hand.

SERVES 2 (MAKES 4 CUPS)

4 cups Bone Broth (page 163)
2 cups shiitake or other mushroom stems, chopped
1 garlic clove, peeled
1 cup chopped fresh parsley, cilantro, or other herb stems
2 tablespoons canned unsweetened coconut milk
2 teaspoons freshly squeezed lemon juice
Pinch of cayenne pepper

(Continues)

(Neglected Veggie Stem Soup Continued)

In a medium-size saucepan, combine the broth, mushroom stems, and garlic. Bring to a simmer over medium-high heat, then lower the heat to maintain a low simmer, cover, and simmer for 30 minutes. Transfer the broth to a blender, add the herb stems, and blend for about 1 minute to break down the stems. Strain back into the pan, pressing on the solids to extract all the green goodness. Add the coconut milk, lemon juice, and cayenne and serve.

Each serving: 23 g protein, 4 g fat, 10 g carbs, 166 calories

TIP: *If you need to reheat the soup, do so gently, or it will lose it vibrant green color. Keep a bag in the freezer that you can collect stems in.*

Ginger Chicken Soup

WITH BONE BROTH and poached chicken on hand, this warming soup is almost instant soup. Or you could poach chicken directly in the soup to double the flavor. To bump this soup up to a meal, add a starchy carb, such as a chopped medium-size sweet potato or ½ cup corn kernels.

SERVES 2 (MAKES ABOUT 4 CUPS)

4 cups Bone Broth (page 163)
1 small carrot, grated
2 garlic cloves, pressed through a garlic press
1 teaspoon ginger juice (see Note)
2 tablespoons coconut aminos
1 cup shredded Poached Chicken (page 178)
1 cup packed baby spinach
1 scallion, white and green parts, thinly sliced

1 serrano or jalapeño chile, cut in half, seeded, and thinly sliced
4 teaspoons freshly squeezed lime juice, or to taste

In a medium-size saucepan, bring the broth to a boil over medium-high heat. Add the carrot, garlic, ginger juice, and coconut aminos, lower the heat to medium, and cook for 1 minute. Add the chicken and spinach and cook to warm through and wilt the spinach. Add the scallion, chile, and lime juice, spoon into bowls, and serve.

Each serving: 42 g protein, 3 g fat, 10 g carbs, 245 calories

- **Add V3**
Double up on the spinach or scallion.

Note: To juice ginger, finely grate a small amount and squeeze the juice from it.

Daily Super Salad

START WITH A base of greens, add some spunk, crunch, kick, umami, and herbal flavor, and a simple salad becomes a Super Salad. Keep things interesting by changing your salad up based on season, whim, or what you've got in the fridge. Choose from the categories below, and go unlimited with your veggies. My favorite is a base of kale and arugula, scallions, cilantro, parsley, shredded carrot, and crumbled grain-free crackers. Remember, it's all about V3: value, volume, veggies! To extend your dressing, serve it in a separate little bowl and dip your fork into it before taking a bite. Enjoy your Super Salad any time of day—for a snack, or with lunch, dinner, or even breakfast!

DRESSING

2 tablespoons Essential Salad Dressing (page 171)

(Continues)

(Daily Super Salad Continued)

GREENS

Arugula
Baby beet greens
Boston lettuce
Butterhead lettuce
Chicory
Dandelion greens
Endive
Escarole
Frisée
Kale leaves
Looseleaf or oakleaf
    lettuce
Mâche
Mesclun
Mizuna
Radicchio
Romaine lettuce
Spinach
Swiss chard leaves
Watercress

CRUNCH

Beets
Bell pepper
Cabbage
Carrots
Celery
Cucumber
Sprouts

SPUNK

Radishes
Red onion
Scallions

KICK

Garlic
Ginger
Grated horseradish
Pickle (page 231)
Sauerkraut (page 174)

UMAMI

Anchovies
Capers
Crunchy Dulse Chips
    (page 231) or dulse
    granules
Mushrooms
Olives
Toasted nori strips
Tomatoes

HERBAL

Basil
Chives
Cilantro
Dill
Mint
Parsley
Rosemary

FRUITY

Apple
Berries
Grapefruit
Grapes
Orange

FATTY (1½ TABLESPOONS PER SALAD)

Almonds
Avocado
Brazil nuts
Cashews
Hazelnuts
Macadamia nuts
Poppy seeds
Pumpkin seeds
Sesame seeds
Sunflower seeds

> ### *Veggies, Front and Center*
>
> Don't confine your veggies to the crisper drawer. Set them front and center in your fridge in glass bowls so you can see them when you open the door. When you keep them within reach, you won't lose track of them and it will be easy to find inspiration for your Daily Super Salad.

Snacks and Treats

Everything Crackers

THESE CRISP AND crunchy crackers are surprisingly easy to make. And they'll save you money and detective work: no more sorting through sometimes confusing ingredients lists to figure out which grain-free brands are actually unprocessed. Save any uneven edges after rolling out the dough; break them up into coarse crumbs to stand in for croutons to toss over soups or salads.

MAKE ABOUT 50 CRACKERS

2 cups almond flour
1½ teaspoons toasted sesame seeds
1½ teaspoons poppy seeds
½ teaspoon sea salt
1 large egg

Preheat the oven to 350°F.

In a food processor, combine the almond flour, sesame seeds, poppy seeds, and ¼ teaspoon of the salt and pulse to combine. Add the egg and

(Continues)

(Everything Crackers Continued)

pulse until the mixture comes together into a crumbly dough. Remove the dough from the food processor and form it into two oval mounds with your hands.

Put one dough mound in the center of a large piece of parchment paper and flatten it slightly with your hands. Cover with a second piece of parchment or a silicone mat and use a rolling pin to roll it out as thinly as possible (see Tip for mastering the rolling technique).

Put the dough setup on a baking sheet and remove the top piece of parchment. Repeat with the remaining dough round, placing it on a second baking sheet. Sprinkle both rounds with the remaining ¼ teaspoon of salt and gently pat the salt so it sticks to the dough. Use a pizza wheel to cut the dough into approximately 1½-inch squares directly on the parchment, trimming the rough edges. Prick each cracker square with the tines of a fork for effect, if you like. Bake until lightly browned, about 15 minutes, then remove from the oven, allow to cool, and separate the crackers. Keep in an airtight container on the counter for up to 1 month.

> **TIP:** To get your dough cracker-thin, try this: After you roll the dough a couple of times, gently lift the top piece of parchment and place it back down. Then, flip the whole thing over, lift the second piece of parchment, and continue rolling. Repeat until you've reached your target thickness. This will keep your dough from sticking to the parchment and enable you to go superthin, just like the crackers you get from a box.

Each serving (2 crackers):
3 g protein, 4 g fat, 3 g carbs, 56 calories

Crunchy Dulse Chips

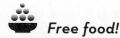 *Free food!*

IF YOU LIKE the taste of bacon (who doesn't?), the salty, smoky flavor of dulse is your sea vegetable of choice. Dulse is full of vitamins, minerals, and antioxidants, and like all sea vegetables, it has more nutrients than plants grown on land. I can't think of a better reason to swap your processed fix for crunchy dulse chips. Eat them out of hand, or top soups or salads with them to make any dish a superdish!

SERVES 6

1 ounce whole leaf dulse

Preheat the oven to 400°F.

Place the dulse on a baking sheet and bake for about 15 minutes, turning every 5 minutes, until crispy. Allow to cool and store on the counter in a covered jar for up to 2 weeks.

> **Each serving:**
> 1 g protein, 0 g fat, 2 g carbs, 12 calories

Traditional Dill Pickles

 Free food!

CRUNCHY, TANGY NATURALLY fermented dill pickles are a cinch to make. The recipe is simply packing cucumbers into a jar, adding dill and garlic, covering the whole thing with salt water, and waiting a week or two for the cucumbers to turn into pickles.

Fermented pickles differ from the ones you buy on the shelf: those are made with vinegar and often sugar and contain no active cultures. Fermented

(Continues)

(Traditional Dill Pickles Continued)

pickles are the real deal! Read more about the life-giving benefits of fermentation on page 93. For this recipe, you will need a 2-quart wide-mouth glass jar and filtered water to make brine, as the chlorine in tap water may affect fermentation.

MAKES 2 QUARTS

1 quart filtered water
2½ tablespoons fine sea salt
1 bunch fresh dill
6 garlic cloves, peeled
2 pounds small to medium-size Kirby or pickling cucumbers

Combine 3 cups of the water and the salt in a small saucepan. Bring to a simmer over medium heat. Set aside, stirring occasionally, until the salt is dissolved. Pour into a jar or glass measuring cup, add the remaining cup of water, and allow to cool completely.

Put the dill and garlic in a 2-quart wide-mouth glass jar, then put the cucumbers on top. Pour enough brine over the cucumbers to cover them, leaving at least 1 inch of space remaining at the top (you may have leftover brine).

Place the jar on a rimmed plate (in case of spills). Fill a jar big enough to fit through the mouth of the pickle jar with water, put the lid on, and place it over the pickles. This serves as your weight to keep the pickles covered in brine. Cover with a clean dish towel and set aside in a cool place away from sunlight to ferment. Check the pickle jar every day and remove the mold with a clean spoon if any develops.

Your pickles will be ready in 1 to 2 weeks, depending on how warm it is in your kitchen and how sour you like them. Cover and refrigerate; the pickles will keep for about 2 months.

Each serving (1 medium-size pickle):
0 g protein, 0 g fat, 2 g carbs, 9 calories

● *Supercharge It!*
- Add spices, such as black or white peppercorns, red pepper flakes, mustard seeds, cumin seeds, coriander seeds, or juniper berries.
- Pickle other vegetables, such as carrots, beets, and green beans; the firmer the veggie, the longer it will take to ferment.

Zucchini and Roasted Yellow Pepper Hummus

ZUCCHINI TAKES THE place of chickpeas to add veggie goodness to your hummus experience. Yellow peppers and turmeric give it a beautiful golden color. Use a carrot stick or Everything Cracker (page 229) for dipping, or thin the hummus with a little water or olive oil and it will do double duty as a salad dressing.

MAKES ABOUT 3 CUPS

1¼ cups raw cashews, soaked in water to cover for 4 hours
1 small zucchini, chopped
2 roasted yellow peppers (see sidebar), chopped
1¼ cups raw cashews, soaked in water to cover for 4 hours
⅓ cup tahini (sesame paste)
3 tablespoons freshly squeezed lemon juice
3 tablespoons extra-virgin olive oil
1 garlic clove, chopped
1 teaspoon sea salt
1 teaspoon paprika
½ teaspoon ground cumin
½ teaspoon ground turmeric
¼ teaspoon freshly ground black pepper

(Continues)

(*Zucchini and Roasted Yellow Pepper Hummus Continued*)

Put the cashews in a medium-size bowl and add hot water to cover by a couple of inches. Cover with a dish towel and leave to soak and soften for at least 1 hour or up to 4 hours. Drain.

Combine all the ingredients in a food processor or blender and process until very smooth, scraping the sides as needed, 3 to 5 minutes. Add a little water if it is too thick. The hummus will keep, covered and refrigerated, for up to 5 days.

Each serving (¼ cup):
4 g protein, 13 g fat, 8 g carbs, 157 calories

- *Swap Out*
Use smoked paprika for a smoky hummus or chipotle chile powder for a smoky, spicy hummus.

- *Neglected Veggie Alert!*
No need to trim the stem and bottom from your zucchini. They'll blend right in!

How to Roast Bell Peppers

ON A GAS STOVETOP:

Set the peppers on the grate directly over a high flame. Using tongs, turn the peppers occasionally until the skin is completely blackened, 7 to 8 minutes.

UNDER THE BROILER:

Set the broiler to HIGH. Place your peppers on a baking sheet and place it directly under the broiler. Using tongs, turn the peppers a few times until the skin is completely blackened, 7 to 8 minutes.

TO PEEL THEM:

As soon as the peppers are blackened, put them in a heatproof bowl and cover with a plate or pot lid. Leave for about 20 minutes to steam, then peel off the skin with your fingers (avoid washing the peppers, as it will rinse off some of the flavor).

TO STORE AND USE:

The peppers will keep refrigerated in an airtight container for up to 5 days. In addition to hummus, you can add them to salads, stir-fries, and scrambles.

Mushroom Jerky

PORTOBELLO MUSHROOMS MARINATED in savory coconut aminos and slowly baked become a veggie version of jerky, a great way of getting in a superfood in volume! These are also great savory topping for your Super Salad (page 227).

SERVES 4

¼ cup coconut aminos
¼ cup cider vinegar
1½ tablespoons extra-virgin olive oil
1 tablespoon dulse flakes
1 teaspoon garlic powder
1 teaspoon onion powder
½ teaspoon freshly ground black pepper
6 portobello mushrooms, sliced ¼ inch thick

In a small bowl, whisk together the coconut aminos, vinegar, oil, dulse, garlic powder, onion powder, and black pepper. Place the mushroom slices in a resealable plastic bag, add the marinade, and toss to coat. Refrigerate for at least 8 hours or up to 12 hours, turning a couple of times to keep the mushrooms evenly marinated.

Preheat the oven to 225°F and line two baking sheets with parchment paper.

Drain the mushrooms from their marinade. Arrange the mushroom slices on the sheets with a little space between each. Bake for 1½ to 2 hours, turning halfway through, until the pieces have completely dried out and have a chewy (not crisp) texture. Remove from the oven and allow to cool completely, then transfer to a container, cover, and store in the refrigerator for up to 1 week.

Each serving: 3 g protein, 5 g fat, 13 g carbs, 113 calories

Almond Protein Bites

WHILE TRYING TO get in protein to fuel our workouts, many of us over-look the fact that most protein bars are filled with less than healthy ingredients and tons of sugar. These little bites get their protein from almonds, sweetness from dates, and raw cacao nibs for chocolaty crunch with each bite. Eat one to refuel your body postworkout, for a midday snack, or to tide you over until dinner.

MAKES 18 BITES (1 BITE PER SERVING)

2 cups pitted dried dates
2 cups almonds
1 cup unsweetened shredded coconut
2 tablespoons coconut oil
1 teaspoon pure vanilla extract
½ teaspoon salt
¼ cup goji berries
⅓ cup raw pumpkin seeds
2 tablespoons raw cacao nibs

Place the dates in a bowl and add warm water to cover. Leave for about 20 minutes for the dates to soften, then drain the water.

In a food processor or high-speed blender, combine the almonds and co-conut and blend until broken down to a powder. Add the dates, oil, vanilla, and salt and blend until well combined. Transfer to a bowl and work in the goji berries, pumpkin seeds, and cacao nibs with your hands. Form into eighteen 1½-inch balls. Place into a container and store in the refrigerator for up to 1 week or in the freezer for up to 2 months.

Each serving: 6 g protein, 14 g fat, 20 g carbs, 214 calories

● *Swap Out*
  • Try dried currants instead of goji berries.
  • Swap sunflower seeds for the pumpkin seeds.

Coconut Chip Trail Mix

TOASTING BRINGS THE natural oils of nuts to the surface, adding crunch and extra-nutty flavor. Toasting your own nuts means you avoid the processed oils and salt typically found in packaged nuts for an upgrade to your trail mix. Many trail mixes are more like dessert, but swapping in cacao nibs keeps the sugar in check while satisfying the chocoholic in you. This is a perfect snack to keep in your purse, backpack, or lunch box.

MAKES 3 CUPS

1 cup raw almonds
½ cup raw walnut or pecan halves
½ cup raw cashews
1 cup unsweetened flaked coconut
⅓ cup raw cacao nibs
¼ cup goji berries
¼ cup raisins

Combine the nuts in a dry, heavy skillet. Place over medium heat and toast, stirring often, until they are lightly browned and toasty smelling, about 5 minutes. Lower the heat if the nuts start to burn. Transfer to a plate to cool. Lower the heat to medium-low, add the coconut, and toast, stirring constantly, until light golden and fragrant, about 2 minutes. Add to the plate of nuts and allow to cool completely.

Combine the nuts, toasted coconut, cacao nibs, goji berries, and raisins in a large bowl or storage container and stir thoroughly to mix.

Each serving (¼ cup):
6 g protein, 16 g fat, 13 g carbs, 209 calories

TIP: Divide the trail mix into individual servings in resealable snack bags to avoid oversnacking.

Banana Nut Muffins

THESE HIGH-PROTEIN MUFFINS are light, moist, and sweetened only with banana to energize you while keeping your blood sugar stable. The recipe doubles easily, so you can eat some now and freeze the rest for later.

MAKES 12 MUFFINS (1 MUFFIN PER SERVING)

3 very ripe bananas, broken into chunks

3 large eggs

1 cup almond flour

½ cup almond or other nut butter, homemade (page 169) or store-bought

3 tablespoons coconut oil, melted and cooled

2 teaspoons ground cinnamon

½ teaspoon baking powder

½ teaspoon baking soda

¼ teaspoon salt

1 teaspoon pure vanilla extract

½ teaspoon almond extract

1 tablespoon slivered almonds

Preheat the oven to 350°F and line a 12-well muffin pan with paper liners.

In a blender, combine the bananas, eggs, almond flour, almond butter, coconut oil, cinnamon, baking powder, baking soda, salt, and vanilla and almond extracts and blend until smooth.

Pour the batter into the muffin cups, filling them almost to the top. Top each muffin with some of the slivered almonds, lightly pressing them into the batter. Bake until lightly browned on top and a toothpick inserted into the center of a muffin comes out clean, 20 to 25 minutes. Allow the muffins to cool in the pan for 10 minutes, then remove them and serve. The muffins will keep, wrapped in plastic wrap, in the refrigerator for up to 5 days or in the freezer for up to 2 months.

(Continues)

(Banana Nut Muffins Continued)

Each serving: 7 g protein, 14 g fat, 13 g carbs, 197 calories

TIP: Buy extra bananas to ripen and freeze so you'll have them on hand for smoothies.

Raw Cacao Fudge

DENSE YET LIGHT, nutty, crunchy, and extra-chocolaty . . . this recipe is everything you want from fudge, minus the processed sugar, dairy, and artificial ingredients! It takes just five minutes to put together, and your efforts are rewarded generously: heart-healthy omega-3 fatty acids from the walnuts, fiber and sugar-free sweetness from dates, and lots of cacao powder to bring the antioxidant content off the charts. And there's no cooking required!

MAKES 36 SQUARES

¾ cup raw cacao powder
2 cups walnuts
2 cups pitted dried dates
2 tablespoons coconut oil, melted
1 teaspoon pure vanilla extract
½ teaspoon sea salt
2 tablespoons raw cacao nibs

Line the bottom of an 8-inch square baking pan with parchment paper.

Place the cacao powder in a food processor. Add the walnuts, dates, coconut oil, vanilla, and salt. Process until the nuts are broken down into small bits and the mixture looks like loose crumbs (not smooth). Test by pressing a bit together with your hands. If it sticks together easily, it's ready to go. If not, pulse it a few more times, but don't go too long or it will turn into a paste. Add the cacao nibs and pulse just to combine.

Press the mixture into the prepared pan. Place in the refrigerator or freezer and chill until firmed up, then use a butter knife to cut into three dozen squares (5 cuts across lengthwise, and then again widthwise). Store, covered, in the refrigerator for up to 2 weeks or in the freezer for up to 4 months.

Each serving (1 square): 1 g protein, 5 g fat, 9 g carbs, 82 calories

Frozen Fig and Cocoa Cheesecake Bites

THESE BITES ARE pure delight! Sweetened with dates and figs and made creamy with cashews and coconut, they are a reward for unprocessing your diet. Store in the freezer until you are ready to enjoy one, then let it thaw for ten minutes (no more) before popping it into your mouth.

MAKES 12 CHEESECAKE BITES

½ cup raw cashews
⅓ cup dried figs
⅓ cup pitted dried dates
3 tablespoons coconut oil
⅓ cup unsweetened canned full-fat coconut cream or coconut milk
3 tablespoons raw cacao powder
¼ teaspoon sea salt
½ teaspoon pure almond extract

Put the cashews in a small bowl and add water to cover by a couple of inches. Trim off the tough tip of the fig stems and put the figs and dates in a separate bowl. Add hot water to cover by a couple of inches. Cover with a dish towel and leave to soak and soften for at least 1 hour or up to 4 hours. Drain.

Line a 12-well mini muffin pan with paper liners.

(Continues)

(*Frozen Fig and Cocoa Cheesecake Bites Continued*)

In a high-speed blender or food processor, combine all the ingredients and process until very smooth, about 3 minutes, stopping to scrape down the sides of the processor bowl if needed. (You'll get the creamiest results from a blender.) Divide the cheesecake "batter" among the paper liners, using 2 tablespoons for each. Smooth the tops with a small rubber spatula or spoon. Place in the freezer and freeze until solid, about 3 hours, then transfer to a resealable plastic freezer bag. The cheesecake bites will keep in the freezer for up to 2 months. Let thaw for about 10 minutes (do not let them thaw completely or they will collapse) before popping one into your mouth.

Each serving: 1 g protein, 7 g fat, 8 g carbs, 104 calories

Strawberries and Coconut Whipped Cream

WHEN YOU EAT a processed foods diet, your taste buds are constantly assaulted with sugar. So, when you eat a naturally sweet food, it no longer tastes very sweet. But when you unprocess your diet, you win back your taste buds, and a fruit becomes a sweet treat once again. Top a bowl of strawberries—or any fruit you like—with a spoonful of coconut whipped cream. Not only will you be amazed at how deliciously sweet fresh fruit is, you'll feel truly satisfied.

SERVES 2

1 pint strawberries, hulled and sliced
4 tablespoons Coconut Whipped Cream (page 181)
Optional toppings: cacao nibs, unsweetened shredded coconut, a
   sprinkle of cinnamon or nutmeg

Divide the strawberries between two bowls. Top with the coconut cream and your choice of toppings and serve.

Each serving (without toppings):
1 g protein, 6 g fat, 12 g carbs, 106 calories

TIP: *Save the stems and hulls from your strawberries and add them to your smoothies. Yes, you can eat them!*

Sixteen Simple Snacks

Nori grabbers: Mix grated carrots and cabbage, sprouts, and julienned cucumber (or whatever veggies you like). Grab a sheet of nori and use it to wrap the vegetables. Dip into No-Peanut Peanut Sauce (page 198) or a mix of 2 tablespoons of coconut aminos, 1 tablespoon of white wine vinegar, and a pinch of red pepper flakes. No nori? No problem—use hearty collard, red cabbage, or kale leaves.

Nutty fruit or veggies slices: Spread nut butter over sliced apple, peach, or celery.

Roasted herb nuts: Heat 1½ teaspoons of extra-virgin olive oil in a medium-size skillet over medium heat. Add 1 cup of raw almonds, cashews, walnuts, or pecans; ½ teaspoon of dried oregano, Italian seasoning, or thyme; and a large pinch of salt and toast for about 5 minutes, until lightly browned all over. Enjoy 1 to 2 tablespoons as part of a weight-loss plan or ¼ cup for maintenance.

Hard- or soft-boiled eggs: Make them as soon as you get home with the carton and store them in the fridge. Voilà, ready-made protein snack when you're hungry!

Frozen grapes: A refreshing way to satisfy your sweet tooth. Pop grapes into a resealable plastic bag and freeze.

(Continues)

(Sixteen Simple Snacks Continued)

Smoked salmon rolls: Roll a slice of smoked salmon inside a strip of cucumber, with a dab of pesto if you like.

A pickle: Make my recipe on page 231, or choose a naturally fermented brand from the refrigerator section to satisfy your craving for salt and your body's need for probiotics.

Coconut butter: Made from blending the whole coconut, it's rich, velvety, and sweet but with a very low sugar content. A spoonful can satisfy a craving for something sweet on the spot!

Cheese and crackers: Spread Everything Crackers (page 229) with Creamy Cashew Cheese (page 170).

Cheesy date: Spread Creamy Cashew Cheese (page 170) inside a pitted date.

Green salsa and crudités: Dip veggie sticks into Green Salsa (page 173). Both nonstarchy vegetables and green salsa are unlimited!

Chili pumpkin seeds: Heat 1½ teaspoons of extra-virgin olive oil in a medium-size skillet over medium heat. Add 1 cup of raw pumpkin seeds, ½ teaspoon of chili powder, and a large pinch of salt and toast for about 5 minutes, until lightly browned all over. Enjoy 1 to 2 tablespoons as part of a weight-loss plan or ¼ cup for maintenance.

Caffeine and cream: Top a cup of coffee or tea with a spoonful of Coconut Whipped Cream (page 181).

Grapefruit brûlée: Run a grapefruit half under the broiler until browned, about 5 minutes.

Spicy cukes: Sprinkle cucumber wedges with salt, chili powder, and a squeeze of lime.

Seaweed snacks: Toasted crisp nori sheets are one packaged snack product I'm in favor of. They satisfy the urge for something salty while infusing your body with the mega nutrients sea vegetables contain. Make sure your seaweed snacks contain no sweeteners or processed oils.

....
Transformation
....

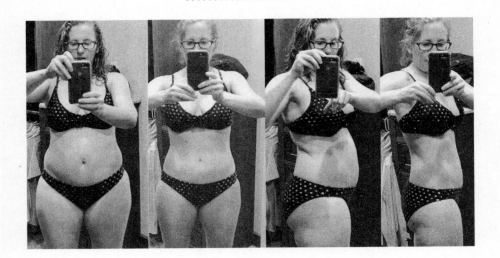

AMANDA

"You Can't Out-Exercise a Bad Diet"

I have struggled with my weight at since I became a mother. My kids are twelve, nine, and four now. I had always been active, but having kids, aging, and not changing my diet to keep up got me 30 pounds overweight. I've tried a lot of things along the way, from paleo to Whole30, and they never worked. Changing my state was what changed everything. Without changing my mind, I couldn't change the rest.

When I joined Natalie's Full Body Reset, I was at my heaviest. A big part of the program for me was figuring out my why and understanding what was stopping me. I lost 6 pounds in six weeks, then I hit a plateau for three or four weeks. At that point in a program, I usually go back to how I ate before, but this time I committed to seeing it through, and then I started to lose weight again.

I always thought of myself as big boned. When I was a teenager, I was a dancer. Everything revolved around weight and I got rail thin. I told myself I didn't want to get too serious about diet, or I'd become too thin again. Through the Aging in Reverse program, I realized that was a self-imposed stop, and in actuality there was no way I'd allow that to happen again.

I'm a busy doctor who doesn't like to cook, but I made time to do this. I followed the plan exactly for ten days, then I did a simplified version after so I didn't have to make three new meals each day. I had already unprocessed my diet, so giving up dairy and grains was doable for me. The results: I felt more energetic and the irritable bowel syndrome I normally suffer from was gone. I had my period halfway through and there was no cramping. I'm on week five as I write this, and I still feel great. I may stay this way the rest of my life! On my last vacation I resisted s'mores, which are usually my downfall. I was feeling so good I didn't want to derail it with something that I knew would make me feel worse in the end. I lost 9 pounds in four weeks and 21 pounds total in the six months I've been working Natalie's programs.

My vision was to be calm and focused because I tend to run around like a crazy person. I've made an effort to be present with my kids. My driving core motivator is my family. I trail run, scuba dive, hike, and ice skate with my three active boys. I love exercising. It's my release and I want to continue to be strong. I want to be able to do all those activities with my kids and their kids, too! I used to think exercise was the driver for the machine, that if you exercise more, you'll lose weight. But you can't out-exercise a bad diet!

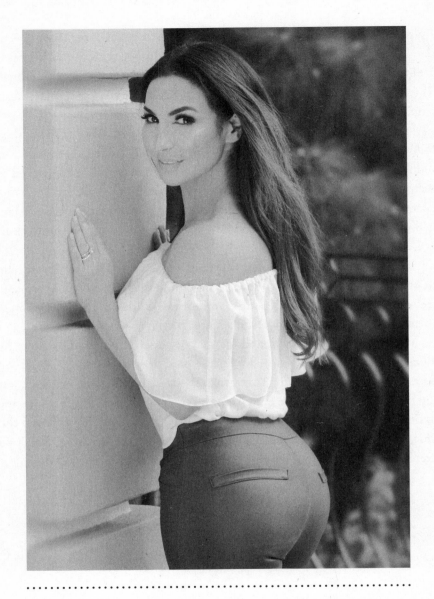

If you want to feel better, you've got to love yourself just as you are. That's the only way lasting change can happen.

PART 3

Love Your Weight

Easier said than done, you may say. But there's no way around it. If you want to feel better, you've got to love yourself just as you are. That's the only way lasting change can happen. Loving your weight opens you up to the big picture of your life, enables you to make changes that last, and completes the Transformation Triangle.

First, I want you to consider this: You weigh what you weigh right now for a reason. The old calories-in, calories-out model of weight is less relevant as you age, so the cause might not be as straightforward as you think. Your body can pack on fat to protect you from food sensitivities, stress, gut imbalances, hormone imbalances, or changes such as those experienced in perimenopause and menopause.

What to do? The first thing I'm going to ask of you is to be kind to yourself. If you start out hating yourself, you'll just be setting yourself up for disappointment. Focus on something you like or love about yourself. For example, *I like the way my calves look; I like my smile.* Think of how you're getting stronger and better all the time. Use what you've learned in Change Your State to engage your mind-set. You've gotten clear on your vision (page 13), you've honed in on your driving core motivator (page 25), you've made a commitment (page 28), and you've connected with the right people (page 42). Plug yourself into gratitude and your whole mood will shift, you will find inspiration, and change will happen.

By setting your goals in motion, you've found inspiration to Plan Your Plate (page 51) and follow through. You're fueling your body with what it really needs. Only then can a workout program truly succeed. Through this empowerment, you will complete the Transformation Triangle. Well done!

First, Get Up!

Before you engage in a new fitness routine, get up off your seat! Sitting can be as damaging to your health as smoking and can sabotage your fat-loss efforts. Going to the gym three or four times a week is amazing, but you need to be moving *throughout* the day, every day. Don't be stationary! Movement is so important to fat loss because it keeps your metabolism revved up. Consider getting a Fitbit for tracking and think of creative ways to get up and get your steps in. Here are a few ideas to get you started:

- Use a stand-up desk or a stability ball instead of a chair.

- Walk around your house or yard when you're on the phone.

- Walk up and down a flight of stairs at the office.

- Walk to a coworker's office rather than e-mailing her.

- Walk at lunch.

- Walk after meals.

- Have a walking meeting with a colleague.

- Walk to work or get off one stop earlier on the bus or subway.

- Put a stepper under your desk.

- Walk while brushing your teeth.

- Meet friends for a walk instead of tea.

- Set reminder alerts on your phone to get up.

- Walk around the track or field while your kids play sports.

- Start a walking group at work or with friends.

Just thirty minutes of walking a day can significantly decrease your chance getting cardiac disease or diabetes (but no need to stop there). Walking can improve your mood and fight off depression, and it can lower overall body weight and decrease body fat. Get up and move daily!

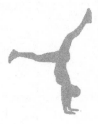

Step 1

Focus on Intensity and Progression

Contrary to what most of us have learned, results don't come from time. Progression and intensity are what will change your body. It doesn't matter whether you worked out for twenty minutes, an hour, or five hours. And there's no magic rep set. If you just go with a number, you're not really in touch with your body. Counting and doing the same mindless movements is dated and does not help you progress. Without progression, muscle mass decreases and you don't see improvement.

Progression means improving and challenging yourself every day. Imagine picking up a plastic bag from the floor. If you can bend down, there's no question you can pick up the plastic bag. Now imagine engaging your core and bracing your glutes to pick up a cement block. That's the force and the attitude with which I want you to go into your workouts. Ask yourself how you can make it more challenging for yourself. Any exercise you add to your routine should be one that you can progressively dial up so you can continue to see results.

Long, drawn-out cardio workouts will not get you to the next level—especially if you are reading or texting when you do it. It's a good start, but body weight exercises will challenge you more, keep you progressing, and raise the intensity.

WHAT DO YOU LOVE ABOUT YOUR BODY?

No matter where you are in reaching your health and fitness goals, you can always find something to love about your body. Start basic, and don't just focus on appearance but, rather, on how your body works. *I can smell my coffee in the morning. I can taste the sweetness of an apple. I can breathe. I can walk. I can move.* Keep going and don't stop until you've filled out a full page.

Now, look over your list and pick something you want to improve. Not *change*, but *improve*. For example, if you love the way your body feels when you stretch, think of ways you can become more flexible. If you are happy with how strong your legs are, think of how you can get them even stronger and more toned. The plan is to improve on what is already there. When you focus on making the good better, other things inevitably will change, too!

Understand the Benefits of Body Weight Exercises

I'm not against going to the gym and doing the circuits if that's what works for you. But when you're lifting weights or using machines, you don't always use the muscles they are intended for, which can cause you to lock down other areas of your body. For example, if you add a heavy weight to a bicep curl, there's a chance you'll engage your lower back and swing your shoulders to get the weight up. That means you're not actually working your bicep muscle to the fullest, which can lead to imbalances and injury.

What I find most effective for my clients is body weight exercise, because it allows them to clearly measure their progression. A push-up is an example of a body weight exercise. The very act of working toward doing even one push-up can be challenging for many. Moving from no push-ups to one push-up, or five or ten, is easily measurable. The same goes for a plank. At first you might not even be able to do a plank for one second, but when you find yourself holding your plank for a minute, you can congratulate yourself because you know just how much you've progressed. Another benefit of body weight exercises: you can do them at home so you don't have to go to a gym!

MOVE EVEN MORE DURING PERIMENOPAUSE AND MENOPAUSE

The more you move, the less weight you'll gain as your hormones change. But unfortunately, the trend is for women to put the brakes on exercise as they get older. Whether you are going through perimenopause or you are looking to lose weight postmenopause, exercising is critical for maintaining a healthy weight—true at any time in life, and now more than ever. Strength training and staying active—keeping your body moving—will help you shed extra pounds and maintain your weight. It's great if you are fit enough to perform vigorous aerobic activities, such as jogging and swimming, but if you aren't, you can start with moderate aerobic activity, such as brisk walking. Any movement is better than nothing! Remember, it's not just about what you do in the gym. Movement counts at any time of day and all the chances you have to move, whether it's taking the stairs, doing a few lunges at your desk, or walking instead of taking a cab a few blocks, will add up to better health. You can start with small, manageable exercise goals and build on those as you get stronger. You'll begin to shed fat and gain muscle, and as you gain muscle, your body's metabolism will speed up and start to burn calories more efficiently. This makes it easier to control your weight.

Although all you learned in Plan Your Plate will help you counteract the effects of menopause, prevention is always better than cure. If you start working on your health and fitness now, it will definitely pay you in the future and you will have fewer chances of weight gain and improved overall health for the long haul.

Don't Just Look Fit, Be Fit

Strive to become functionally fit. *Functionally fit* means your whole body moves and flows together. There are no imbalances or areas that don't work well. You are free of aches and pains and you move at ease. Your core is at the base of functional fitness. When that midsection area—your abs, back, and hip flexors to some extent—is strong and working properly, it should take the bulk of force from your exercise movements and keep you from feeling pain in your lower back, neck, and joints.

Looking fit means you have lost fat and pumped up your muscles in all the right places, but that doesn't necessarily mean your body feels good and is moving without pain. Many fitness buffs look great but are in pain on a daily basis. That is the opposite of being functionally fit!

When you start focusing on being functionally fit, you'll start to appreciate the benefits of exercise that you don't see on the outside. Regular exercise has been linked to lower risk of chronic disease, lower levels of stress and anxiety, improvements in cognition and brain function, and increased life span. Resistance training has been shown to lower white matter lesion volume in the brain, which means lower risk of dementia, and exercising can also improve memory, which can counteract the brain fog we can experience later in life (see page 129). Staying active can also help you sleep better at night, reduce fatigue and anxiety, improve self-esteem, and even reduce hot flashes during menopause.

Another benefit of exercise, particularly weight training exercise, is that it can strengthen your bones. We know bone density is a crucial topic as we age (see page 130) and resistance training can help counteract the reductions in bone density we typically experience during menopause. Bone strength is vital as we get older to help prevent fractures and other injuries. You'll also see gains in muscle when you start exercising (at a time of life when we typically lose muscle mass!).

While weight loss and toned muscles are certainly important, they are just two pieces of the puzzle when it comes to exercise benefits. Countless studies have linked consistent exercise to improved quality of life, and this goes hand in hand with functional fitness. Yes, you will look better, but you will also *feel* better and *function* better as you step up your exercise game.

Find the Right Exercises for You

Most of us spend a lot of time doing the *wrong* exercises. For example, if just hearing the word *plank* makes your wrists hurt, then you may be doing it wrong (I'll show you the correct way on page 270). If an exercise leaves your joints or back hurting, you are likely doing it wrong. You should feel your muscles working, but you shouldn't feel pain. And you should feel energized and strong after your workouts. Doing the right exercises for you in the right way is the only way to dial up the intensity and keep progressing. When you have injuries or long-standing imbalances, you don't move your body in the way it should be moving. Read on to get your body working the right way!

WORK TOWARD STRONGER, NOT SKINNY

Working toward *skinny* and focusing on a size or number on the scale is subjective, unempowering, and discouraging. Working toward *stronger* is measurable, positive, and possible!

Step 2

10 Daily Mindful Movements for Strength, Flexibility, and a Pain-Free Body

The following ten movements are designed to reset your body and get you moving the way you are meant to move. They will help prevent injury, reduce and even reverse inflammation and pain, strengthen your core, and build up the small neglected and often overlooked muscles in your body. And they help get you get through your workouts pain free! Do them every day in conjunction with whatever exercise routine you enjoy. Note that you'll need a foam roller, and one of the exercises has a bench option. For floor work, you'll need a yoga mat or towel.

Diaphragm Breathing

Did you know that there are healthy and unhealthy ways to breathe? If you've ever been to a yoga class, at some point the teacher probably instructed you to "breathe deeply into your belly." This is intuitively relaxing, but there's more to it. How we breathe affects everything we do in life—how we carry ourselves, how we react to stress, and even the quality of our workouts.

What that yoga teacher was referring to is known as diaphragm breathing. The diaphragm is the dome-shaped muscle found at the base of our lungs and is the most efficient muscle for breathing. Our abdominal muscles help move the diaphragm and give us more power to empty our lungs. Here are some of its benefits:

- Floods the body with fresh oxygen

- Stimulates a calming response

- Rejuvenates the circulatory system

- Decreases our demand for oxygen

- Stimulates brain activity

- Neutralizes the fear response

- Slows down our pulse

- Allows us to use less energy to breathe

In our overburdened lives, we have lost track of our breath. We no longer naturally breathe through our diaphragm—the natural way to breathe—and instead take shallow breaths from our chest. This gets us more stressed, and our neck and chest muscles take on the greater burden of breathing. And it can leave the diaphragm weakened and flattened and working less efficiently.

How to know whether you are breathing correctly? Place your hands on your belly and breathe as you normally breathe. Notice whether your belly is pulling in or pushing out when you take a breath. If your belly pulls in on the inhale, your breath will be shallow, letting the air only enter the top part of your lungs. Let's change that!

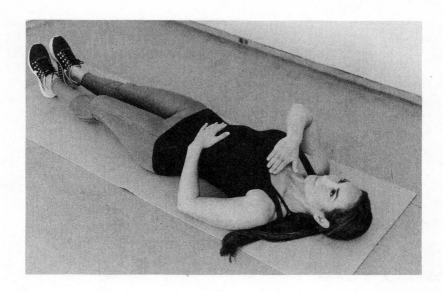

1. Diaphragm Breathing

1. **Sit comfortably in a chair** or on the ground (with a cushion to support you, if needed) with your spine lengthened. Relax your head, neck, and shoulders.

2. **Put your hands on your** belly and inhale so your stomach moves out against your hand. The hand on your chest should remain as still as possible. Feel your body expand. If your breath doesn't make it to your belly at first, don't worry. Continue to practice, and eventually it will come.

3. **Place one hand on your** upper chest and the other just below your rib cage. This will allow you to feel your diaphragm move as you breathe.

4. **Tighten your stomach muscles, letting** them fall inward as you exhale, and feel your body contract. Keeping the hand on your upper chest as still as possible, let all the air from your lungs release.

5. **Start again. Repeat this breath** for 5 minutes daily and incorporate it into your stretches.

▶ **Variation:** *You may also practice this breath lying down with your knees bent and a pillow under your head for support if needed.*

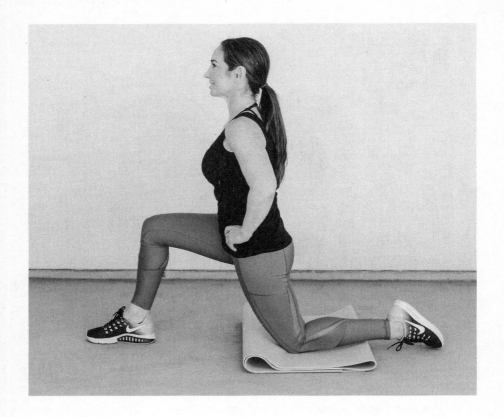

2. *Stretches*

Hip Flexor Stretch

Prolonged sitting leads to tight hip flexors, which can lead to lower back pain and muscles spasms. This exercise directly counters the sitting position so as to correctly release your hip flexors.

Get down on your knees and bring your right foot forward so your right knee is at a 90-degree angle from the floor. Put a mat or other padding under your knees, if needed. Squeeze your left glute and hamstring. Bring your trunk forward very slightly for a mini stretch, but don't dig all the way in, to avoid straining your lower back. Lift your left arm up and over to lean into it to increase the stretch. Hold for 30 seconds, then repeat on the other side.

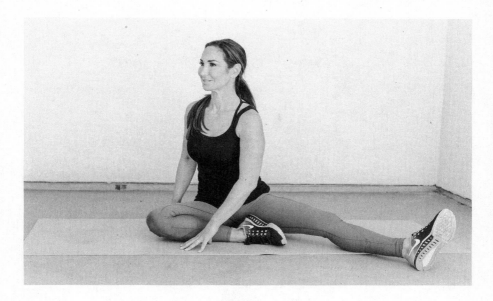

QL Stretches

The quadratus lumborum (QL) is located in the lower part of your back on either side of your spine. A tight QL can cause hip and back pain, so it's important to stretch it out. Note: Your level of flexibility isn't the important part; the key is to get a little hamstring stretch and to really get into that QL area.

Sit down with your left leg forward and your right leg bent with the sole of your foot touching your left thigh. You may bend your left leg slightly to avoid straining your back. Line yourself up to your right leg first, then turn and twist over your left leg. Hold for 1 to 2 minutes, then repeat on the other side.

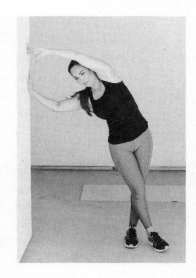

▶ **Variation:** *Use a wall as a base. Hold onto the wall with your right hand and, with your knees slightly bent, cross your right leg over your left. Lift your left arm over your body to touch the wall and lean into your QL. Repeat on the other side.*

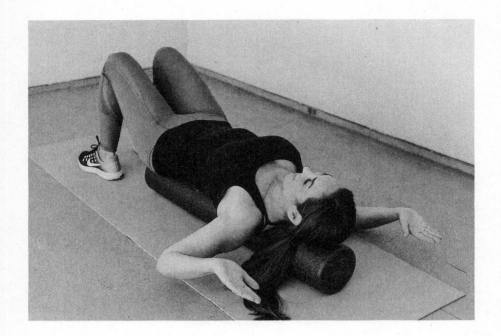

Chest Opener

Sitting in front of a computer pushes our shoulders and head forward. This exercise counters that.

Lie down on a foam roller with the roller under the length of your back. Put your arms out with your elbows bent. The goal is not to get your arms all the way down but to really open your chest. Hold for at least 1 minute and breathe deeply.

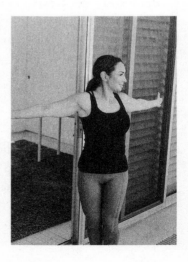

▶ **Variation:** *If you don't have a foam roller, stand in front of a door frame. Hold onto the side of the door opening with your right hand and stretch your left arm all the way back to open your chest. Hold for at least 1 minute, then repeat on the other side.*

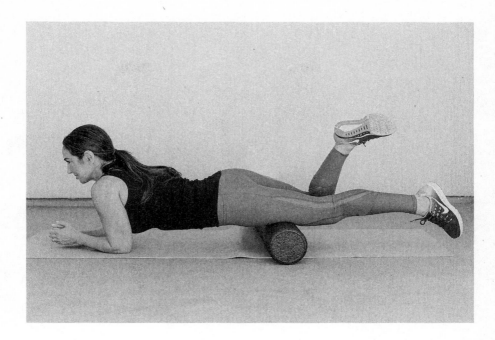

Quad Foam Rolling

Most people, especially women, are quad dominant. (Quads are the muscles on the front of your thighs.) By foam rolling those quads, we turn them off so as to activate our glutes.

Lie facedown and put a foam roller under your quads. Start rolling, moving and twisting to get at your whole quad and hip flexor area. Focus on any tight spots and knots and work those a bit more. Continue for at least 1 minute.

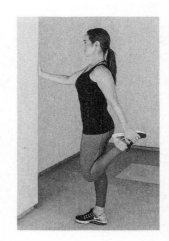

▶ **Variation:** *If you don't have a foam roller, stand up with your core tight. Bend your left knee and grab your left foot from behind you and stretch. Hold onto a wall, if you need to. Repeat on the other side.*

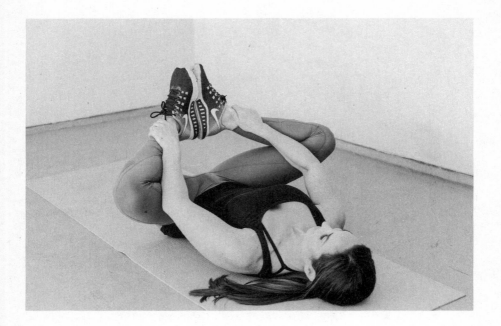

Butterfly Stretch

This stretch opens your inner thighs, stretches your hip flexors, and strengthens your core.

Lie on your back with your lower back pressed into the ground. Put the soles of your feet together with your knees out. Engaging your core, gently press down on your thighs and hold for 30 seconds.

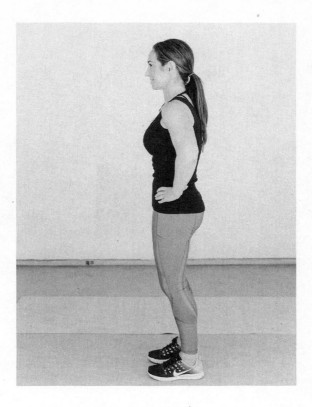

3. Core Bracing

This exercise will feel great in your back, glutes, and abs. Do it often throughout the day—while you're doing dishes, for a micro break from sitting at your desk, and so on.

Stand up straight and perform a rocking motion with your pelvis to find your neutral spine (this is when everything is in alignment and you are neither super arched nor super tucked under). Engage your glutes and abs and pull your ribs down and shoulders back to stack your spine. When you're bracing correctly, you can really feel it in your abs. Do this for 10 seconds as many times a day as you can.

▶ **Variation:** *You can also do this sitting or lying down with your knees bent and feet flat on the floor.*

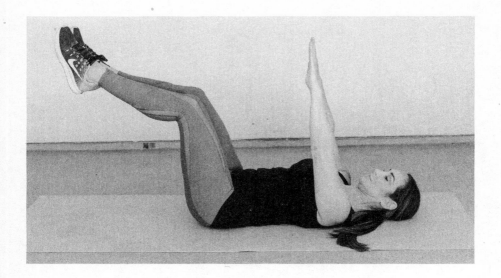

4. Deadbugs

This exercise strengthens your hip flexors, works your abdominal muscles, and engages your core. A neutral spine is critical. It is easy not to engage your core and not press your lower back into the ground. Be aware!

Lie down on your back and lift both legs with your knees bent. Press your lower back into the ground to get at a neutral spine. Feel your abs engage. A good way to test for neutral spine is to try to slip your hand between your lower back and the ground. If your hand fits, you are arching rather than in neutral. Hold this position for a minimum of 1 minute.

▶ **To make it more challenging,** *bring your legs a little lower while continuing to engage your core, then alternate touching your feet down to the ground. Make sure your lower back is still pressed to the floor; if you begin to arch, don't lower your legs as much.*

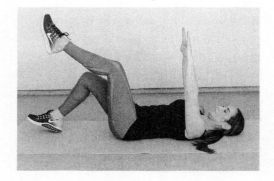

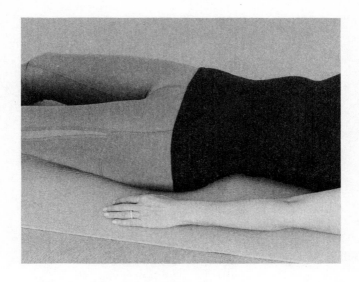

5. Glute Squeezes

Practicing isolating and activating your glutes helps to remedy quad dominance.

Lie down on your back with your legs straight out and core braced. One at a time, squeeze your glutes to get them to fire. Start with 1 minute and work up to 2 minutes.

▶ **Variation:** *You can do this standing or sitting in a chair as well.*

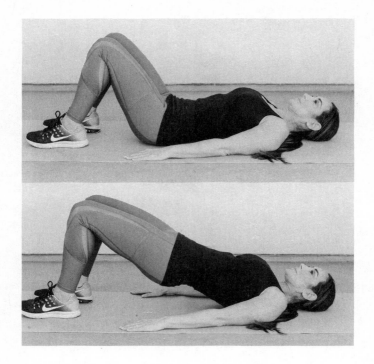

6. Glute Bridges

This is another one for activating your glutes and countering quad dominance.

Lie down on your back with your knees bent and your feet on the ground, with your arms straight next to you, palms down, and with your fingers and toes pointed forward. With your core braced, lift your hips while engaging your glutes and hamstrings and driving through your heels. Drive through your booty and do not swing through your back. Go up and down for 1 minute, or squeeze and hold for up to 1 minute.

▶ **Bench Variation:** *Lie down with your back on the edge of the bench. Either cross your arms over your chest or have them open across the bench. Concentrate on pushing through your heels and keep your whole upper body working as one unit. Lower yourself down and up. It's okay if your toes come off the ground. Make sure to squeeze your booty and hamstrings as you work. It's quality over quantity, and it's fine to go slow.*

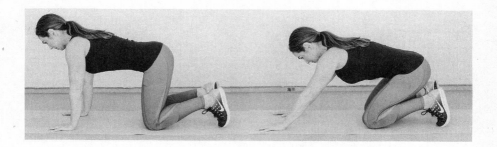

7. Pain-Relieving Squats

A piece of PVC pipe keeps you in alignment to let you know you're doing your squats the right way.

To prepare for your squats, get down on your hands and knees with your toes on the floor and your hands under your shoulders and rock back and forth, driving through your heels and activating your glutes. Continue for 1 minute.

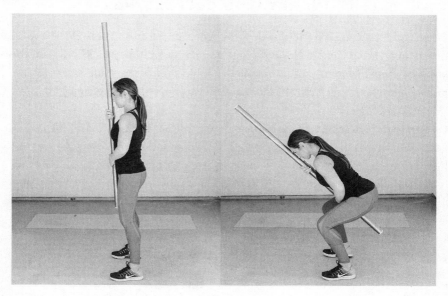

To do your squats, set a piece of PVC pipe (or a stick) against the center of your chest and down through to your pubic bone. Go from standing to squat, up and down, for 30 seconds.

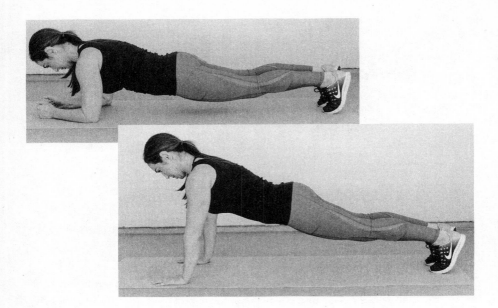

8. Planks (the correct way)

Plank is the best exercise to develop your core, and a strong core gives you support in everything you do. **Note: A plank should never hurt your shoulders, forearms, or back.** *In fact, your lower back should feel great while you're doing a plank. If you feel pain in any of those areas, you aren't in the correct form.*

Get on your forearms and toes. Push up and squeeze your glutes. Make sure to keep your stomach up with your pelvis tucked in and your lower back flat. Now here is where many of us make a mistake: we arch our back because we think it looks flattering or we don't know better. That is the *incorrect* way to do a plank. The correct way to do a plank is to straighten that natural C-curve so your back is flat. Next, try to move from your forearms to your hands and hold it there. Start at 30 seconds and work up to 3 minutes.

▶ **Modification:** *Tap a knee down to make it easier.*

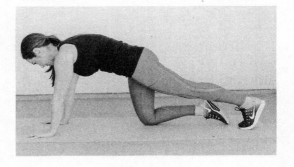

9. Push-ups

Push-ups are the ultimate upper body movement and are effective for toning and defining. Not only do they build upper arm and chest strength, but they also are great for strengthening your core. All of these versions of the push-up start in plank position.

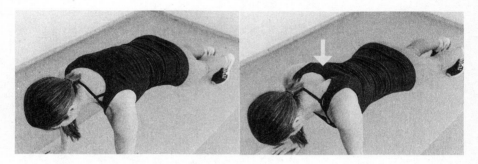

▲ **Scapula:** From a plank position with arms wide, make slight movements with your scapula.

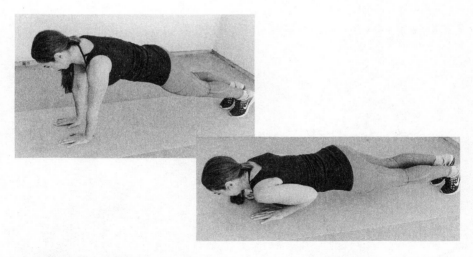

▲ **Triceps:** Still in a plank position, bring your hands in a little so your elbows are close to your sides. Go all the way down and back up, making sure your elbows don't wing out.

(Push-ups Continue)

(*Push-ups Continued*)

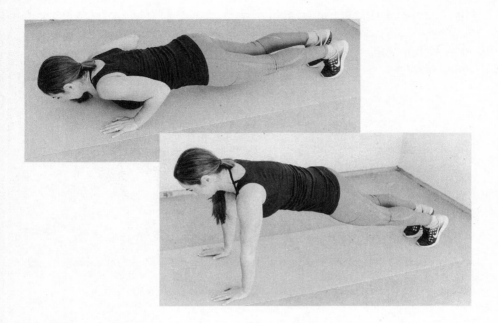

▲ **Chest:** Bring your hands wide again and go all the way up and down.

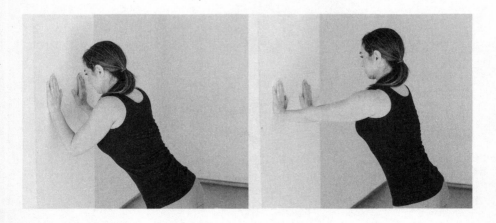

▲ **Modification:** *Bend your knees or do your push-ups against a wall.*

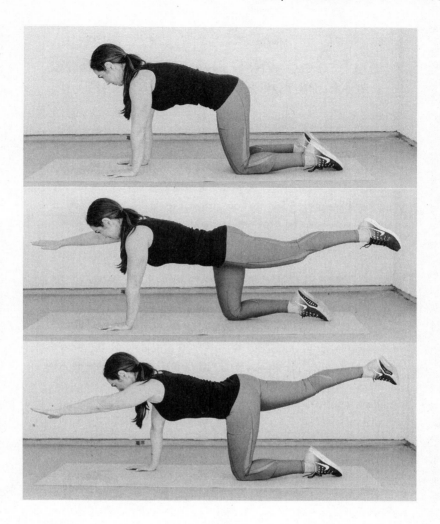

10. Bird Dogs

This is a great overall restorative movement. It helps warm up your core, lower back, glutes, and upper body, and it's great for balance and stability.

Get down on your hands and knees with your toes on the floor and your hands under your shoulders. With your glutes squeezed and your core tight, lift your right leg and straighten it out behind you. Lift your left arm and straighten it out in front of you. Switch sides and continue alternating sides for 1 minute.

WHAT TO DO WHEN AN INJURY OR ILLNESS KEEPS YOU FROM WORKING OUT

Working out is the foundation of my career, and also it's an outlet that makes me productive in everything else I do. However, I've had many times in my life when an injury got in my way of my workouts. After recent surgery, I was under doctor's orders not to work out for at least six weeks. As you can imagine, this was very hard for me! But while I was preparing for my comeback, I took notes on what I did so I could share these tips for returning stronger with you:

1. Become Your Own Diet Doctor

When an injury or illness gets in your way of exercising, your diet becomes even more important. This is the time when you'll start storing fat if you don't watch what you eat. I suggest you up your protein (while slightly lowering your carbs and fat so you aren't increasing total calories) so you don't lose muscle as quickly and eat more fruits and vegetables to feed your body the nutrients it needs to recover quickly. I know it's tempting, but don't sit on the couch and start eating chips, candy, and soda, because that is guaranteed to make you feel worse!

2. Get Creative in Your Activity

Take inventory of what you can do. Can you stretch? Can you walk? Can you move at all? Can you stand instead of sitting while you're working? If you have a lower-body injury, try doing something with your upper body, and so on. After my surgery, I was told to limit my exercise to walking, so that's what I did. Figure out what you can do and do it. Every little bit counts.

3. Stay Committed to Your Mind-set

Take this time to plan and create a new vision for what you want to do when you get back on track. Research new types of workouts.

Watch those self-imposed stops (see page 21). Make a new vision board (see page 13) and start making new goals.

4. Fill the Void

You know, that to-do list and pile of stuff you've been putting off or never get to because so many other things come first, such as your workouts. You'll feel more empowered when you get back to your routine.

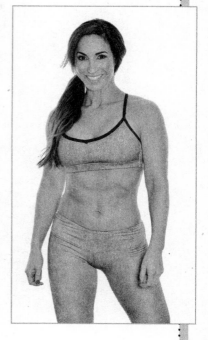

EMBRACE AN ATHLETE MENTALITY

Have you ever watched a professional or elite athlete train? If you have, you know what I'm talking about. You know she is fueling her body with good nutrition for great performance and is not starving herself when the scale doesn't read the ridiculously low number so many of us beat ourselves up over daily.

Think like an athlete would in whatever you do—in the gym, at work, and in every part of your life. Go all in 100 percent of the time. Don't just go through the motions but do the full intensity of the exercises so you can keep progressing. Move your body every day in a way that's healthy for you, and give it everything you've got. An athlete learns to adjust her mind-set to achieve new goals. She has no quit drive. She's mindful of her body and her mental state. Apply what you learned in Change Your State (see page 11) to act as if you're already there—as if failure is not an option. Start doing everything it takes!

························
Transformation
························

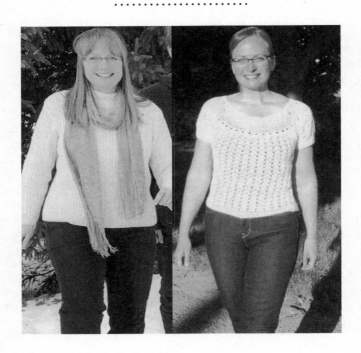

TERRI
"I Love the Holistic Approach"

Growing up, I was a figure skater and I was always fit. I never had a weight issue. But then I injured my back, and things started to change. I packed on the pounds and started yo-yo dieting, which messed with my metabolism. I got depressed and let a lot of things go. So, after I made the decision to be healthy, I put together a vision board with images of nice hair, fitness people, six-pack abs, and vacations. That kept me on track and accountable. I made a plan to succeed. Once I changed my mind-set, I was able to really focus on the food. With Natalie, it's not just about weight loss but how you look at the world. I call it the Natalie Jill lifestyle.

I lost 35 pounds from working Natalie's programs and wanted to lose 10 more. When I started Aging in Reverse, I had already given up most grains and other starchy carbs. The biggest challenge for me was eliminating whey protein power from my smoothies because the whey makes the smoothies creamy. But when I made my first Super Green Smoothie, I was relieved to find that it was creamy and awesome! I started using collagen protein and some avocado or ½ banana to make my smoothies creamy, and I was surprised at how much I liked them. The most unique recipe was the Carrot Cake Colada Smoothie—it's the most spices I've ever put into a smoothie in my life. I love all the recipes, and I was never hungry. Without grains and dairy, my digestion was better and I had less bloating. My mood was great and I had lots of energy. My husband jumped on board with me, which made it that much easier. I'm fifty and I don't have any hormonal issues related to perimenopause. A lot of people comment that I look a lot younger since I lost weight, and my daughter says my skin looks better. In the ten days, I lost 4 pounds and 5 inches. But it's the whole picture that's really changed. Natalie taught me the why and how of being mentally and physically healthy. I love the holistic approach!

Final Words

The exercises in the final chapter are not a full workout plan; rather, they are designed to help you recover, heal, and get ready to move your body. There's no one right way to start or continue a workout plan, but there are two words to remember: *intensity* and *progression*. Move your body daily. Keep going forward and keep challenging yourself. Think longer, more frequently, and upping the intensity. For example, if you want to walk, start with a couple of blocks, then from there you might push it to a mile and increase the pace and how often you commit to walking. It's the same with body weight exercises: think of how you can start using your body in a way that you are progressing every day. Take the 10 Daily Mindful Movements on pages 259 to 273 as a base and move forward from there. And my website, www.nataliejillfitness .com, offers a variety of body-weight DVDs to help set a plan for yourself.

You're getting in shape, you've taken unprocessed to the next level, and aging in reverse has become a reality for you. When you're in maintenance mode (pages 135 to 138), the time may come when you feel so good that you don't remember how you felt before, and you revert to old ways of eating. Or your motivation is lagging, you feel as though you're just getting by, and you don't think you have it in you to continue full force. That's the time to come full circle and revisit that State section (starting on page 11). While the recipes will fill your belly and please your palate, your state is the secret ingredient. Revisit your vision, your driving core motivator, and your goals. Dig deep and shift that state of mind. You are always one decision away from the *right* decision. Focus on your potential, not your setbacks. You've got this!

The Recipes

Acknowledgments

First off, I want to thank Renée Sedliar and the team at Da Capo Press for their support and amazing energy and commitment as we turned this vision into a reality. Writing a book is an amazing experience and a very involved process. This book would not have been possible without the professional guidance form the following people (in no particular order): Leda Scheintaub, Julie Grimes, Celeste Fine, John Mass, Jaidree Braddix, Jenn LaVardera, and Noel Daganta.

In addition to the professionals that made this book come to fruition, there were mentors and friends and family that inspired and encouraged me along the way. We are the *sum* of who we surround ourselves with and I am so lucky to have such an amazing tribe around me!

Thank you to my team in and out of NJF for supporting my vision. Liana Hunt, Nicole Fryer, Lauren Reid, Jess Jacobson, Katrina Lacbungan, Justin Schenck, and Mindy Marinos: I am so grateful to you.

Thank you to the most *amazing* mentors, coaches, and friends: James Wedmore, Frank and Natalia Kern, Vince DelMonte, Michael Strasner, Chris Lee, Jenna and Brad Ballard, and Torey Wolford. Thank you Shanda Sumpter and Ash Ghandahari for seeing the greatness in *me* and standing for me to go on the road of personal development. To the *entire* classes of ALA SD9, HCL1, HCL5, and MLP2: I am forever grateful to you for breaking me through my *own* self-imposed stops and being my family in transformation.

Thank you, Dr. Choll Kim, for repairing me when I had lost hope and for the following people for helping me discover and recover: Reece Jensen, the MoveU team of Mike Wasilisin and Andrew Dettelbach, Jen Esquire, Charleston Cruz, Marie Lemkul, and Todd Durkin!

Thank you to my *girls* who lift me up, are examples, and contribute so greatly to this world! Natalia Kern, Natalie Minh, Lori Harder, Chalene

Johnson, Allison Maslan, Lori Taylor, and so many more! You inspire me to "Be" *more*!

Thank you to my "sister from another mister" Deirdre Gonzalez, for being a sounding board and a truest friend. I am so lucky to have you in my life and her husband, Jeremy Gonazlez (my daughter's dad), for being a stand for excellence.

To my *tribe:* my ladies—Members of my Full Body Reset, VIP breakthrough weekend girls, coaching clients, and members of my NJFitSquad!—I love you more than you will ever know. Thank *you* for being a mirror for me daily and so open and committed. Your breakthroughs are *results* of my vision!

To the listeners and GUESTS on my Podcast: "Leveling Up: Creating Everything from Nothing" thank you for motivating me DAILY to continue reaching for more.

To my mom and dad, who taught me as a child that anything and everything is possible if we can envision it.

A *special* huge heartfelt thank-you to my soulmate, my best friend, my *rock,* and my *husband,* Brooks Hollan. I love you more than words can do justice. This book would have never come to fruition without you.

To my daughter Penelope, who reminds me daily what it means to live in the moment and be playful and free. You both are my world. Thanks for encouraging me to pursue my dreams always. *I love you both* so much.

References

Body

Perimenopause to Menopause

"Perimenopause: Rocky Road to Menopause," Harvard Health Publishing (June 2009, updated August 24, 2018), https://www.health.harvard.edu/womens-health /perimenopause-rocky-road-to-menopause.

Menopause and Weight Gain

Ekta Kapoor, Maria L. Collazo-Clavell, MD, and Stephanie S. Faubion, MD, "Weight Gain in Women at Midlife: A Concise Review of the Pathophysiology and Strategies for Management," *Mayo Clinic Proceedings* 92, no. 10 (October 2017): 1552–1558, https://www.mayoclinicproceedings.org/article/S0025 -6196(17)30602-X/fulltext.

Lisa M. Neff et al., "Core Body Temperature Is Lower in Postmenopausal Women Than Premenopausal Women: Potential Implications for Energy Metabolism and Midlife Weight Gain," *Cardiovascular Endocrinology* 5, no. 4 (December 2016): 151–154, https://www.ncbi.nlm.nih.gov/pmc/articles/PMC5242227/.

S. R. Davis et al., "Understanding Weight Gain at Menopause," *Climacteric* 15, no. 5 (2012): 419–429, https://www.tandfonline.com/doi/full/10.3109/13697137.2012 .707385.

Sleep and Weight Gain

American Thoracic Society, "Sleeping Less Linked to Weight Gain," ScienceDaily (May 2006), www.sciencedaily.com/releases/2006/05/060529082903.htm.

Metabolism

A. Coyoy, C. Guerra-Araiza, and I. Camacho-Arroyo, "Metabolism Regulation by Estrogens and Their Receptors in the Central Nervous System Before and After Menopause," *Hormone and Metabolic Research* 48, no. 8 (August 2016): 489–496, https://www.ncbi.nlm.nih.gov/pubmed/27392117.

Inflammation

Anne M. Minihane et al., "Low-Grade Inflammation, Diet Composition and Health: Current Research Evidence and Its Translation," *British Journal of Nutrition* 114, no. 7 (October 14, 2015): 999–1012, https://www.ncbi.nlm.nih.gov/pmc/articles /PMC4579563/.

"Foods That Fight Inflammation," Harvard Women's Health Watch (June 2014, updated August 13, 2017), https://www.health.harvard.edu/staying-healthy /foods-that-fight-inflammation.

Hyokjoon Kwon and Jeffrey E. Pessin, "Adipokines Mediate Inflammation and Insulin," *Frontiers in Endocrinology* 4, no. 71 (June 2013), https://www.ncbi.nlm .nih.gov/pmc/articles/PMC3679475/.

Paul DiCorleto, PhD, "Why You Should Pay Attention to Chronic Inflammation," Cleveland Clinic (October 14, 2014), https://health.clevelandclinic.org/why-you -should-pay-attention-to-chronic-inflammation/.

Menopause and Brain Fog

Emily G. Jacobs et al., "Impact of Sex and Menopausal Status on Episodic Memory Circuitry in Early Midlife," *Journal of Neuroscience* 36, no. 39 (September 28, 2016): 10163–10173, http://www.jneurosci.org/content/36/39/10163.

Emily G. Jacobs and Jill M. Goldstein, "The Middle-Aged Brain: Biological Sex and Sex Hormones Shape Memory Circuitry," *Current Opinion in Behavioral Sciences* 23 (October 2018): 84–91, https://www.sciencedirect.com/science/article/pii /S2352154617302061.

Pauline M. Maki and Victor W. Henderson, "Cognition and the Menopause Transition," *Menopause* 23, no. 7 (July 2016): 803–805, https://insights.ovid.com /pubmed?pmid=27272226.

Stephanie V. Koebele et al., "Cognitive Changes Across the Menopause Transition: A Longitudinal Evaluation of the Impact of Age and Ovarian Status on Spatial Memory," *Hormones and Behavior* 87 (January 2017): 96–114, https://www .sciencedirect.com/science/article/pii/S0018506X16302446.

Menopause and Fatigue/Sleep

Asuka Hirose et al., "Effect of Soy Lecithin on Fatigue and Menopausal Symptoms in Middle-Aged Women: A Randomized, Double-Blind, Placebo-Controlled Study," *Nutrition Journal* 17, no. 4 (January 2018), https://nutritionj.biomedcentral.com /articles/10.1186/s12937-018-0314-5.

Joyce Walsleben, RN, PhD, "Menopause and Insomnia," National Sleep Foundation, (2018), https://sleepfoundation.org/ask-the-expert/menopause-and-insomnia.

Menopause and Gut Health

Angélica T. Vieira, Paula M. Castelo, Daniel A. Ribeiro, and Caroline M. Ferreira, "Influence of Oral and Gut Microbiota in the Health of Menopausal Women," *Frontiers in Microbiology* 8, no. 1884 (September 28, 2017), https://www.frontiersin.org/articles/10.3389/fmicb.2017.01884/full.

Menopause and Bone Health

H. K. Väänänen and P. L. Härkönen, "Estrogen and Bone Metabolism," *Maturitas* 23, suppl. (May 1996): S65–S69, https://www.ncbi.nlm.nih.gov/pubmed/8865143.

Jane A. Cauley, "Bone Health After Menopause," *Current Opinion in Endocrinology, Diabetes and Obesity* 22, no. 6 (December 2015): 490–494, http://journals.sagepub.com/doi/abs/10.2217/WHE.14.40.

Jane A. Cauley, "Estrogen and Bone Health in Men and Women," *Steroids* 99, part A (July 2015): 11–15, https://www.sciencedirect.com/science/article/pii/S0039128X14003031.

Jonathan D. Schepper et al., "Probiotics in Gut-Signaling," *Advances in Experimental Medicine and Biology* 1033 (2017): 225–247, https://www.ncbi.nlm.nih.gov/pmc/articles/PMC5762128/.

Stress

"Why Stress Causes People to Overeat," Harvard Mental Health Letter (February 2012, updated July 18, 2018), https://www.health.harvard.edu/newsletter_article/why-stress-causes-people-to-overeat.

Telomeres

Marta Crous-Bou et al., "Mediterranean Diet and Telomere Length in Nurses' Health Study: Population Based Cohort Study," *BMJ* 349 (2014), https://www.bmj.com/content/349/bmj.g6674.

P. D. Loprinzi, J. P. Loenneke, and E. H. Blackburn, "Movement-Based Behaviors and Leukocyte Telomere Length Among US Adults," *Medicine and Science in Sports and Exercise* 47, no. 11 (November 2015): 2347–2352, https://www.ncbi.nlm.nih.gov/pubmed/25970659.

Food

Cacao

David O. Kennedy and Emma L. Wightman, "Herbal Extracts and Phytochemicals: Plant Secondary Metabolites and the Enhancement of Human Brain Function," *Advances in Nutrition* 2, no. 1 (January 2011): 32–50, https://academic.oup.com/advances/article/2/1/32/4591639.

Rafael Franco, Ainhoa Oñatibia-Astibia, and Eva Martínez-Pinilla, "Health Benefits of Methylxanthines in Cacao and Chocolate," *Nutrients* 5, no. 10 (2013): 4159–4173, http://www.mdpi.com/2072-6643/5/10/4159/htm.

Sandra M. Hannum and John W. Erdman Jr., "Emerging Health Benefits from Cocoa and Chocolate," *Journal of Medicinal Food* 3, no. 2 (2004): 73, https://www.liebertpub.com/doi/abs/10.1089/109662000416276?journalCode=jmf.

Canola Oil
Guy Crosby, "Ask the Expert: Concerns About Canola Oil," Harvard T. H. Chan School of Public Health Nutrition Source (April 13, 2015), https://www.hsph.harvard.edu/nutritionsource/2015/04/13/ask-the-expert-concerns-about-canola-oil/.

Carbohydrates and Depression
Jame E. Gangwisch et al., "High Glycemic Index Diet as a Risk Factor for Depression: Analyses from the Women's Health Initiative," *American Journal of Clinical Nutrition* 102, no. 2 (August 1, 2015): 454–463, http://ajcn.nutrition.org/content/early/2015/06/24/ajcn.114.103846.abstract.

Bone Loss and Added Sugars
Leo Tjäderhane and Markku Larmas, "A High Sucrose Diet Decreases the Mechanical Strength of Bones in Growing Rats," *Journal of Nutrition* 128, no. 10 (October 1, 1998): 1807–1810, https://academic.oup.com/jn/article/128/10/1807/4723108.

Cruciferous Vegetables
"Cruciferous Vegetables and Cancer Prevention," National Cancer Institute (June 7, 2012), https://www.cancer.gov/about-cancer/causes-prevention/risk/diet/cruciferous-vegetables-fact-sheet.

Gluten
Anna Sapone et al., "Spectrum of Gluten-Related Disorders: Consensus on New Nomenclature and Classification," *BMC Medicine* 10, no. 13 (February 7, 2012), https://bmcmedicine.biomedcentral.com/articles/10.1186/1741-7015-10-13.

Grażyna Czaja-Bulsa, "Non Coeliac Gluten Sensitivity—A New Disease with Gluten Intolerance," *Clinical Nutrition* 34, no. 2 (April 2015): 189–194, https://www.clinicalnutritionjournal.com/article/S0261-5614(14)00218-0/fulltext.

Karin de Punder and Leo Pruimboom, "The Dietary Intake of Wheat and Other Cereal Grains and Their Role in Inflammation," *Nutrients* 5, no. 3 (March 12, 2013): 771–787, http://www.mdpi.com/2072-6643/5/3/771/htm.

Lorete M. S. Kotze et al., "Impact of a Gluten-Free Diet on Bone Mineral Density in Celiac Patients," *Spanish Journal of Gastroenterology* 108, no. 2 (February 2016): 84–88, http://scielo.isciii.es/scielo.php?script=sci_arttext&pid=S1130-0108201 6000200006.

T. Kemppainen et al., "Bone Recovery After a Gluten-Free Diet: A 5-Year Follow-up Study," *Bone* 25, no. 3 (September 1999): 355–360, https://www.thebonejournal .com/article/S8756-3282(99)00171-4/abstract.

Natural Remedies for Menopause

N. Farhana Mohd Fozi, M. Mazlan, A. Nazrun Shuid, and I. Naina Mohamed, "Milk Thistle: A Future Potential Anti-osteoporotic and Fracture Healing Agent," *Current Drug Targets* 14, no. 14 (December 2013): 1659–1666, https://www.ingenta connect.com/content/ben/cdt/2013/00000014/00000014/art00005.

Nicole A. Brooks et al., "Beneficial Effects of Lepidium meyenii (Maca) on Psychological Symptoms and Measures of Sexual Dysfunction in Postmenopausal Women Are Not Related to Estrogen or Androgen Content," *Menopause* 15, no. 6 (December 2008): 1157–1162, https://journals.lww.com/menopausejournal /Abstract/2008/15060/Beneficial_effects_of_Lepidium_meyenii_Maca _on.24.aspx.

Seung Min Oh et al., "Ethanolic Extract of Dandelion (Taraxacum mongolicum) Induces Estrogenic Activity in MCF-7 Cells and Immature Rats," *Chinese Journal of Natural Medicines* 13, no. 11 (November 2015): 808–814, https://www.science direct.com/science/article/pii/S1875536415300844.

Protein

J. C. Lovejoy, C. M. Champagne, L. de Jonge, H. Xie, and S. R. Smith, "Increased Visceral Fat and Decreased Energy Expenditure During the Menopausal Transition," *International Journal of Obesity* 32, no. 6 (June 2008): 949–958, https://www.ncbi.nlm.nih.gov/pmc/articles/PMC2748330/.

Probiotics

Alicia L. Muhleisen and Melissa M. Herbst-Kralovetz, "Menopause and the Vaginal Microbiome," *European Menopause Journal* 91 (September 2016): 42–50, https: //www.maturitas.org/article/S0378-5122(16)30124-4/abstract?code=mat-site.

Carol S. Johnston and Cindy A. Gaas, "Vinegar: Medicinal Uses and Antiglycemic Effect," *Medscape General Medicine* 8, no. 2 (2006): 61, https://www.ncbi.nlm.nih .gov/pmc/articles/PMC1785201/.

Dase Hunaefi, "Effect of Fermentation on Antioxidant Properties of Red Cabbages," *Food Biotechnology* 27, no. 1 (2013): 66–85, https://www.tandfonline.com/doi /abs/10.1080/08905436.2012.755694.

Eun Kyoung Kim et al., "Fermented Kimchi Reduces Body Weight and Improves Metabolic Parameters in Overweight and Obese Patients," *Nutrition Research* 31, no. 6 (June 2011): 436–443, https://www.sciencedirect.com/science/article /pii/S027153171100114X.

Huey-Shi Lye, Chiu-Yin Kuan, Joo-Ann Ewe, Wai-Yee Fung, and Min-Tze Liong, "The Improvement of Hypertension by Probiotics: Effects on Cholesterol, Diabetes, Renin, and Phytoestrogens," *International Journal of Molecular Sciences* 10, no. 9 (August 2009): 3755–3775, http://www.mdpi.com/1422-0067/10/9 /3755/htm.

M. de Vrese, "Health Benefits of Probiotics and Prebiotics in Women," *Menopause International* 15, no. 1 (March 2009): 35–40, https://www.ncbi.nlm.nih.gov /pubmed/19237621.

Marta Caretto, Andrea Giannini, Eleonora Russo, and Tommaso Simoncini, "Preventing Urinary Tract Infections After Menopause Without Antibiotics," *European Menopause Journal* 99 (May 2017): 43–46, https://www.maturitas.org /article/S0378-5122(17)30058-0/abstract?code=mat-site.

Nilgün H. Budak et al., "Functional Properties of Vinegar," *Journal of Food Science* 79, no. 5 (May 2014): R757–R764, https://onlinelibrary.wiley.com/doi/abs/10.1111 /1750-3841.12434.

T. D. Swartz, F. A. Duca, T. de Wouters, Y. Sakar, and M. Covasa, "Up-regulation of Intestinal Type 1 Taste Receptor 3 and Sodium Glucose Luminal Transporter-1 Expression and Increased Sucrose Intake in Mice Lacking Gut Microbiota," *British Journal of Nutrition* 107, no. 5 (March 2012): 621–630, https://www.ncbi.nlm .nih.gov/pubmed/21781379.

Vitamin D

Consuelo H. Wilkins et al., "Vitamin D Deficiency Is Associated with Low Mood and Worse Cognitive Performance in Older Adults," *American Journal of Geriatric Psychiatry* 14 no. 12 (December 2006): 1032–1040, https://www.sciencedirect .com/science/article/pii/S1064748112608902.

Rebecca E. S. Anglin, Zainab Samaan, Stephen D. Walter, and Sarah D. McDonald, "Vitamin D Deficiency and Depression in Adults: Systematic Review and Meta-analysis," *British Journal of Psychiatry* 202, no. 2 (February 2013): 100–107, https://www.cambridge.org/core/journals/the-british-journal-of-psychiatry

/article/vitamin-d-deficiency-and-depression-in-adults-systematic-review-and
-metaanalysis/F4E7DFBE5A7B99C9E6430AF472286860.

Fats and Brain

Dany Arsenault, Carl Julien, Chuck T. Chen, Richard P. Bazinet, and Frédéric Calon,
"Dietary Intake of Unsaturated Fatty Acids Modulates Physiological Properties of
Entorhinal Cortex Neurons in Mice," *Journal of Neurochemistry* 122, no. 2 (May
2012): 427–443, https://onlinelibrary.wiley.com/doi/abs/10.1111/j.1471-4159
.2012.07772.x.

Julie A. Dumas et al., "Dietary Saturated Fat and Monounsaturated Fat Have
Reversible Effects on Brain Function and the Secretion of Pro-inflammatory
Cytokines in Young Women," *Metabolism* 65, no. 10 (October 2016): 1582–1588,
https://www.ncbi.nlm.nih.gov/pmc/articles/PMC5023067/.

Bone Broth

B. O. Rennard et al., "Chicken Soup Inhibits Neutrophil Chemotaxis in Vitro," *Chest*
118, no. 4 (2000): 1150–1157, https://www.ncbi.nlm.nih.gov/pubmed/11035691.

Artificial Sweeteners

Jotham Suez et al., "Artificial Sweeteners Induce Glucose Intolerance by Altering the
Gut Microbiota," *Nature* 514 (October 9, 2014): 181–186, https://www.nature
.com/articles/nature13793.

M. Yanina Pepino, Courtney D. Tiemann, Bruce W. Patterson, Burton M. Wice, and
Samuel Klein, "Sucralose Affects Glycemic and Hormonal Responses to an Oral
Glucose Load," *Diabetes Care* 36, no. 9 (September 2013): 2530–2535, https:
//www.ncbi.nlm.nih.gov/pubmed/23633524.

Shanna Frisch, "Artificial Sweeteners and Weight Gain: Fighting or Feeding the
Obesity Epidemic?" *Science Journal of the Lander College of Arts and Sciences* 9,
no. 2 (2016): 167–173, https://touroscholar.touro.edu/sjlcas/vol9/iss2/9/.

Susan E. Swithers, "Artificial Sweeteners Produce the Counterintuitive Effect of
Inducing Metabolic Derangements," *Trends in Endocrinology & Metabolism* 24,
no. 9 (September 2013): 431–441, https://www.sciencedirect.com/science/article
/pii/S1043276013000878.

Diet Soda and Migraines

L. C. Newman and R. B. Lipton, "Migraine MLT-down: An Unusual Presentation of
Migraine in Patients with Aspartame-Triggered Headaches," *Headache* 41, no. 9
(October 2001): 899–901, https://www.ncbi.nlm.nih.gov/pubmed/11703479.

Rajendrakumar M. Patel, Rakesh Sarma, and Edwin Grimsley, "Popular Sweetener Sucralose as a Migraine Trigger," *Journal of Head and Face Pain* 46, no. 8 (August 22, 2006): 1303–1304, https://onlinelibrary.wiley.com/doi/abs/10.1111/j.1526 -4610.2006.00543_1.x.

R. B. Lipton, L. C. Newman, J. S. Cohen, and S. Solomon, "Aspartame as a Dietary Trigger of headache," *Headache* 29, no. 2 (February 1989): 90–92, https: //www.ncbi.nlm.nih.gov/pubmed/2708042?dopt=Abstract.

Shirley M. Koehler and Alan Glaros, "The Effect of Aspartame on Migraine Headache," *Journal of Head and Face Pain* 28, no. 1 (February 1988): 10–14, https://onlinelibrary.wiley.com/doi/pdf/10.1111/j.1365-2524.1988.hed2801010.x.

Gluten-Opioid Connection

Leo Pruimboom and Karin de Punder, "The Opioid Effects of Gluten Exorphins: Asymptomatic Celiac Disease," *Journal of Health, Population and Nutrition* 33, no. 24 (2015), https://www.ncbi.nlm.nih.gov/pmc/articles/PMC5025969/.

Dairy-Opioid Connection

H. Teschemacher, G. Kochm, and V. Brantl, "Milk Protein-Derived Opioid Receptor Ligands," *Biopolymers* 4, no. 2 (1997): 99–117, https://www.ncbi.nlm.nih.gov /pubmed/9216246.

Soy

Fang Fang Zhang et al., "Dietary Isoflavone Intake and All-Cause Mortality in Breast Cancer Survivors: The Breast Cancer Family Registry," *Cancer* 123, no. 11 (March 6, 2017): 2070–2079, https://onlinelibrary.wiley.com/doi/abs/10.1002/cncr .30615.

Moshe Shike et al., "The Effects of Soy Supplementation on Gene Expression in Breast Cancer: A Randomized Placebo-Controlled Study," *Journal of the National Cancer Institute* 106, no. 9 (September 1, 2014), https://academic.oup.com/jnci/article /106/9/dju189/907784.

Mushrooms

Ashok Kumar Panda and Kailash Chandra Swain, "Traditional Uses and Medicinal Potential of Cordyceps sinensis of Sikkim," *Journal of Ayurveda and Integrative Medicine* 2, no. 1 (2011): 9–13, https://www.ncbi.nlm.nih.gov/pmc/articles /PMC3121254/.

In-Kyoung Lee, Young-Sook Kim, Yoon-Woo Jang, Jin-Young Jung, and Bong-Sik Yun, "New Antioxidant Polyphenols from the Medicinal Mushroom Inonotus obliquus," *Bioorganic & Medicinal Chemistry Letters* 17 (2007): 6678–6681, https://pdfs.semanticscholar.org/5896/5748a13bd43bd5253128bb7a3422fa 8226d8.pdf.

Lishuai Ma, Haixia Chen, Peng Dong, and Xueming Lu, "Anti-inflammatory and Anticancer Activities of Extracts and Compounds from the Mushroom Inonotus obliquus," *Food Chemistry* 139, no. 1–4 (August 2013): 503–508, https://www.sciencedirect.com/science/article/pii/S0308814613000526.

Mi Ja Chung, Cha-Kwon Chung, Yoonhwa Jeong, and Seung-Shi Ham, "Anticancer Activity of Subfractions Containing Pure Compounds of Chaga Mushroom (Inonotus obliquus) Extract in Human Cancer Cells and in Balbc/c Mice Bearing Sarcoma-180 Cells," *Nutrition Research and Practice* 4, no. 3 (2010): 177–182, https://www.synapse.koreamed.org/Synapse/Data/PDFData/0161NRP/nrp-4-177.pdf.

Myung-Ja Youn et al., "Chaga Nushroom (Inonotus obliquus) Induces G0/G1 Arrest and apoptosis in Human Hepatoma HepG2 Cells," *World Journal of Gastroenterology* 14, no. 4 (January 28, 2008): 511–517, https://www.ncbi.nlm.nih.gov/pmc/articles/PMC2681140/.

Xiaoshuang Dai et al., "Consuming Lentinula edodes (Shiitake) Mushrooms Daily Improves Human Immunity: A Randomized Dietary Intervention in Healthy Young Adults," *Journal of the American College of Nutrition* 34, no. 6 (2015): 478–487, https://www.tandfonline.com/doi/abs/10.1080/07315724.2014.950391?journalCode=uacn20.

Collagen

Kristin L. Clark et al., "24-Week Study on the Use of Collagen Hydrolysate as a Dietary Supplement in Athletes with Activity-Related Joint Pain," *Current Medical Research and Opinion* 24, no. 5 (2008): 1485–1496, https://www.tandfonline.com/doi/abs/10.1185/030079908x291967.

Maryam Borumand and Sara Sibilla, "Daily Consumption of the Collagen Supplement Pure Gold Collagen® Reduces Visible Signs of Aging," *Clinical Interventions in Aging* 9 (2014): 1747–1758, https://www.ncbi.nlm.nih.gov/pmc/articles/PMC4206255/.

Omega-3 Fatty Acids

Artemis P. Simopoulos, "An Increase in the Omega-6/Omega-3 Fatty Acid Ratio Increases the Risk for Obesity," *Nutrients* 8, no. 3 (March 2016): 128, https://www.ncbi.nlm.nih.gov/pmc/articles/PMC4808858/.

Goodarz Danaei et al., "The Preventable Causes of Death in the United States: Comparative Risk Assessment of Dietary, Lifestyle, and Metabolic Risk Factors," *PLoS Medicine* 6, no. 4 (2009), https://journals.plos.org/plosmedicine/article?id=10.1371/journal.pmed.1000058.

J. C. Maroon and J. W. Bost, "Omega-3 Fatty Acids (Fish Oil) as an Anti-inflammatory: An Alternative to Nonsteroidal Anti-inflammatory Drugs for

Discogenic Pain," *Surgical Neurology* 65, no. 4 (2006): 326–331, https://www.ncbi
.nlm.nih.gov/pubmed/16531187.

Organic

Allison Aubrey, "Is Organic More Nutritious? New Study Adds to the Evidence,"
NPR: The Salt (February 18, 2016), https://www.npr.org/sections/thesalt
/2016/02/18/467136329/is-organic-more-nutritious-new-study-adds
-to-the-evidence.

M. Baranski et al., "Higher Antioxidant and Lower Cadmium Concentrations and
Lower Incidence of Pesticide Residues in Organically Grown Crops: A Systematic
Literature Review and Meta-analyses," *British Journal of Nutrition* 112, no. 5
(September 14, 2014): 794–811, https://www.ncbi.nlm.nih.gov/pubmed
/24968103.

Sea Vegetables

Marcel Jaspars and Florence Folmer, "Sea Vegetables for Health," *Food & Health
Innovation* (February 2013), https://www.pacificharvest.co.nz/wp-content/uploads
/2016/07/Sea-Vegetables-for-Health.pdf.

Se-Kwon Kim and Yong-Xin Li, "Medicinal Benefits of Sulfated Polysaccharides from
Sea Vegetables," *Advances in Food and Nutrition Research* 64 (2011): 391–402,
https://www.sciencedirect.com/science/article/pii/B9780123876690000302.

Yan-Jun Xu et al., "Health Benefits of Sea Buckthorn for the Prevention of
Cardiovascular Diseases," *Journal of Functional Foods* 3, no. 1 (January 2011):
2–12, https://www.sciencedirect.com/science/article/pii/S1756464611000028.

Spices

Adriana M. Ojeda-Sana, Catalina M. van Baren, Miguel A. Elechosa, Miguel A. Juárez,
and Silvia Moreno, "New Insights into Antibacterial and Antioxidant Activities of
Rosemary Essential Oils and Their Main Components," *Food Control* 31, no. 1
(May 2013): 189–195, https://www.sciencedirect.com/science/article/pii
/S0956713512005221.

C. Gupta et al., "Comparative Study of Cinnamon Oil and Clove Oil in Some Oral
Microbiota," *Acta Bio Medica* 82, no. 3 (2011): 197–199, http://mattioli1885
journals.com/index.php/actabiomedica/article/view/1729.

Ganapathy Saravanan, Ponnusamy Ponmurugan, Machampalayam Arumugam Deepa,
and Balasubramanian Senthilkumar, "Anti-obesity Action of Gingerol: Effect on
Lipid Profile, Insulin, Leptin, Amylase and Lipase in Male Obese Rats Induced by
a High-Fat Diet," *Journal of the Science of Food and Agriculture* 94, no. 14 (2014):
2972–2977, https://onlinelibrary.wiley.com/doi/abs/10.1002/jsfa.6642.

Jia Zheng et al., "Dietary Capsaicin and Its Anti-obesity Potency: From Mechanism to Clinical Implications," *Bioscience Reports* 37, no. 3 (June 30, 2017), https: //www.ncbi.nlm.nih.gov/pmc/articles/PMC5426284/.

Mark Moss and Lorraine Oliver, "Plasma 1,8-Cineole Correlates with Cognitive Performance Following Exposure to Rosemary Essential Oil Aroma," *Therapeutic Advances in Psychopharmacology* 2, no. 3 (June 2012): 103–113, https: //www.ncbi.nlm.nih.gov/pmc/articles/PMC3736918/.

N. C. C. Silva and A. Fernandes Júnior, "Biological Properties of Medicinal Plants: A Review of Their Antimicrobial Activity," *Journal of Venomous Animals and Toxins including Tropical Diseases* 16, no. 3 (2010): 402–413, http://www.scielo.br /pdf/jvatitd/v16n3/a06v16n3.pdf.

S. P. Malu, G. O. Obochi, E. N. Tawo, and B. E. Nyong, "Antibacterial Activity and Medical Properties of Ginger," *Global Journal of Pure and Applied Sciences* 15, no. 3 (2009): 365–368, http://www.dirtydoglovers.com/wp-content/uploads/2012 /07/research.pdf.

Samir Malhotra and Amrit Pal Singh, "Medicinal Properties of Ginger (Zingiber officinale Rosc.)," *Indian Journal of Natural Products and Resources* 2, no. 6 (2003): 296–301, http://nopr.niscair.res.in/handle/123456789/12292.

Xuesheng Han and Tory L. Parker, "Anti-inflammatory, Tissue Remodeling, Immunomodulatory, and Anticancer Activities of Oregano (Origanum vulgare) Essential Oil in a Human Skin Disease Model," *Biochimie Open* 4 (June 2017): 73–77, https://www.sciencedirect.com/science/article/pii/S2214008517300068.

Yogeshwer Shukla and Madhulika Singh, "Cancer Preventive Properties of Ginger: A Brief Review," *Food and Chemical Toxicology* 45, no. 5 (May 2007): 683–690, https://www.sciencedirect.com/science/article/pii/S027869150600322X.

Yue Zhou et al., "Natural Polyphenols for Prevention and Treatment of Cancer," *Nutrients* 8, no. 8 (August 2016): 515, https://www.ncbi.nlm.nih.gov/pmc /articles/PMC4997428/.

Turmeric

Keith Singletary, "Turmeric: An Overview of Potential Health Benefits," *Nutrition Today* 45, no 5 (2010): 216–225, https://journals.lww.com/nutritiontodayonline /Abstract/2010/09000/Turmeric_An_Overview_of_Potential_Health_Benefits .8.aspx.

S. Bengmark and A. Gil, "Plant-Derived Health—The Effects of Turmeric and Curcuminoids," *Hospitalaria* 24, no. 3 (2009): 273–281, http://discovery .ucl.ac.uk/1313416/.

Exercise

Barbara Sternfeld et al., "Efficacy of Exercise for Menopausal Symptoms: A Randomized Controlled Trial," *Menopause* 21, no. 4 (April 2014): 330–338, https://www.ncbi.nlm.nih.gov/pmc/articles/PMC3858421/.

Mei-Ling Yeh, Ru-Wen Liao, Chin-Che Hsu, Yu-Chu Chung, and Jaung-Geng Lin, "Exercises Improve Body Composition, Cardiovascular Risk Factors and Bone Mineral Density for Menopausal Women: A Systematic Review and Meta-analysis of Randomized Controlled Trials," *Applied Nursing Research* 40 (April 2018): 90–98, https://www.sciencedirect.com/science/article/pii/S0897189716303640.

N. Bolandzadeh et al., "Resistance Training and White Matter Lesion Progression in Older Women: Exploratory Analysis of a 12-Month Randomized Controlled Trial," *Journal of the American Geriatrics Society* 63, no. 10 (October 2015): 2052–2060, https://www.ncbi.nlm.nih.gov/pubmed/26456233.

Patrick J. O'Connor, Matthew P. Herring, and Amanda Caravalho, "Mental Health Benefits of Strength Training in Adults," *American Journal of Lifestyle Medicine* 4, no. 5 (2010), http://journals.sagepub.com/doi/abs/10.1177/1559827610368771.

Tom G. Bailey et al., "Exercise Training Reduces the Acute Physiological Severity of Post-menopausal Hot Flushes," *Journal of Physiology* 594, no. 3 (2016): 657–667, https://physoc.onlinelibrary.wiley.com/doi/pdf/10.1113/JP271456.

Wolfgang Kemmler, Klaus Engelke, Jürgen Weineck, Johannes Hensen, and Willi A. Kalender, "The Erlangen Fitness Osteoporosis Prevention Study: A Controlled Exercise Trial in Early Postmenopausal Women with Low Bone Density—First-Year Results," *Archives of Physical Medicine and Rehabilitation* 84, no. 5 (May 2003): 673–682, https://www.archives-pmr.org/article/S0003-9993(02)04908-0/abstract.

Index

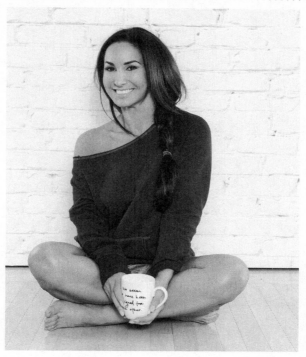

NATALIE JILL is a fat-loss expert turned high performance coach. She helps people across the globe reach their health, business, and life goals by empowering them to level up and create everything from nothing.

Natalie left a very successful career in corporate America to follow her passion with health and personal development.

As a licensed Master Sports Nutritionist, fat-loss expert, and functional fitness trainer, Natalie leveraged the power of the Internet and in a short amount of time was able to help hundreds of thousands of people worldwide get in shape and be their best selves.

In the process, she created a globally recognized brand with well over 2.5 million social media followers worldwide, and created an online business that has consistently generated seven figures a year and has been recognized by *Forbes* and Greatist for two years running as one of the top health and wellness influencers in the world. She is frequently asked about her age (as of this writing, 47) and how she appears to be aging in reverse. Natalie Jill is also the creator and host of the top-ranking podcast "Leveling Up: Creating Everything from Nothing."

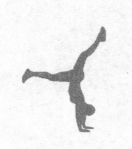